PENGUIN BOOKS

THE NATURAL DIET

Andrew Lockie received his MB, Ch.B. from Aberdeen University, and studied homeopathy at the Royal London Homoeopathic Hospital in 1973–4. He is currently a homeopathic physician in private practice at Guildford, Surrey, and is a founder member of the Homeopathic Physician Teaching Group. His publications are *The Family Guide to Homeopathy*, *The Women's Guide to Homeopathy* and *The Complete Guide to Homeopathy*. Andrew lives in Surrey and his interests include playing the guitar and carpentry.

Janette Marshall is an award-winning writer specializing in the relationship between food and health. As a journalist Janette was editor of *BBC Good Health* magazine, deputy editor of *BBC Good Food* and has been a regular contributor to national newspapers and magazines, including the *Sunday Times* and the *Independent*. Her book, *Eat for Life Diet*, laid to rest the myth that experts cannot agree on what constitutes healthy eating, and has been used by lay readers and health professionals for the last five years. Her popular cookbook, *Fast Food for Vegetarians*, is also available in Penguin. Janette lives in London with her husband and daughter. She enjoys cooking, wine tasting, the theatre, fell walking and keeping fit.

The Natural Diet

Lose Weight with Homeopathy

DR ANDREW LOCKIE
& JANETTE MARSHALL

PENGUIN BOOKS

PENGUIN BOOKS

Published by the Penguin Group
Penguin Books Ltd, 27 Wrights Lane, London w8 5tz, England
Penguin Books USA Inc., 375 Hudson Street, New York, New York 10014, USA
Penguin Books Australia Ltd, Ringwood, Victoria, Australia
Penguin Books Canada Ltd, 10 Alcorn Avenue, Toronto, Ontario, Canada m4v 3b2
Penguin Books (NZ) Ltd, 182–190 Wairau Road, Auckland 10, New Zealand

Penguin Books Ltd, Registered Offices: Harmondsworth, Middlesex, England

First published 1997
10 9 8 7 6 5 4 3 2 1

Set in 11.5/14 pt Monotype Bembo
Typeset by Rowland Phototypesetting Ltd, Bury St Edmunds, Suffolk
Printed in England by Clays Ltd, St Ives plc

Dedicated to M. who showed me the real source of my hunger and thirst and how to truly satisfy them. Also to Babs, Dave, Kirsty, Allie and Sandy for their love and support.

And thanks to Dennis and Mary Thomson for their help and advice.

Andrew Lockie

Both authors would also like to thank Sarah Lutyens.

Contents

1 The Natural Appetite 1

2 Balancing Your Diet with Homeopathy 20

3 An Appetite for Healthy Eating 30

4 The Natural Diet 54

5 Problem Solving 104

6 Finding Your Homeopathic Food Type 120

7 The Natural Diet Maintenance Plan 140

Recipes 148

Selected Bibliography 168

Useful Addresses 172

Index 178

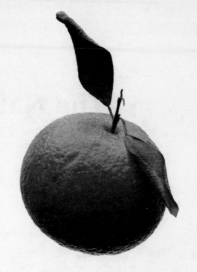

Chapter 1
The Natural Appetite

'Now good digestion wait on appetite,
And health on both!'
  (Macbeth, III, iv, 38)

Why did you last eat? Not *what* or *when* did you last eat, but *why*? Was it because you were hungry, or because someone offered you something you felt obliged to eat? Was it out of habit, or because you were seeking comfort from food?

Our appetite for food is essential to our survival; we need to eat to live. Some of us live to eat. Eating should be one of life's greatest pleasures. The trouble is, eating today can be fraught with difficulties. Many factors disrupt our natural appetite, resulting in extremes such as the current epidemic of obesity and the current fashion for dieting to achieve often unobtainable body images.

We want to guide you through the maze of modern difficulties so that you can eat and enjoy a wide range of tasty foods that will promote health and vitality – and correct your weight problems.

Overweight? Blame it on your Stone Age appetite

Until recently in man's six-million-year history, food has been in short or uncertain supply for many people. To survive, man has needed to eat whenever food was available. Our natural instinct is still to feast at every available opportunity. The difficulty is that this instinct, together with our natural appetite for sugary and fatty foods, is inappropriate today when most of us have sedentary lifestyles and take too many opportunities to eat snacks and meals.

Our craving for high-calorie, sugary and fatty foods evolved in the Stone Age when such foods were scarce and precious. Now that we are frequently exposed to these foods, our appetite leads us to overeat, because natural selection has had neither the need nor the time to adapt our sweet tooth or desire for fats to today's lifestyle.

Genetically, our appetite is still suited to hunting and gathering, and not to fatty diets, cars, central heating and the labour-saving environment in which we now live. The result is an increasing number of overweight people who are biologically defenceless against their weight problems. Our appetites are so sensitive to negative energy balance (i.e., when we are burning more calories than we are eating) that we tend to over-compensate and eat too much. Sadly, we lack an inbuilt compensatory drive against overeating. Appetite is far less sensitive to positive energy balance (i.e., when we consume more calories than we need) and is easily overridden by other pressures, which we will discuss and supply strategies for overcoming.

More weighty problems ahead

The truth is our present-day body was shaped through millions of years of natural selection and adaptation to suit a Stone Age, hunter-gatherer environment. Our love for fatty foods and a sedentary lifestyle is increasing the risk of heart disease, strokes, diabetes, cancer and arthritis. A glance at the table opposite shows how far away from our natural appetite we have moved in the West.

We are eating too much fatty and sugary food and not enough starchy food (bread, potatoes, pasta, rice and other grains). Eating less fat helps weight control and health.

Twenty-five per cent of all British women and 20 per cent of men are predicted to meet the clinical definition of obesity by the year 2005. At the moment, more than 50 per cent of British men and 45 per cent of British women are overweight. If current trends continue unchecked in the USA, the entire population will be obese by the year 2230!

The growing problem of obesity might seem hard to believe when you consider that 30 per cent of women and 20 per cent of men are dieting at any one time. The fact is, while dieting might make you

Percentage of energy obtained from different food components of different human groups

	Hunter gatherers	Peasant agriculturalists	Western societies
Fat (%)	15–20	10–15	40+
Sugar (%)	0	5	20
Carbohydrate (%) (starchy food)	50–70	60–75	25–30
Protein (%)	15–20	10–15	12
Salt (grams/day)	1	5–15	10
Fibre (grams/day)	40	60–120	20

(*Diet, nutrition and the prevention of chronic diseases*, World Health Organisation, 1990)

temporarily slimmer, 95 per cent of people regain the lost weight after a diet, which proves that diets do not work in the long term.

For some people, the fact that our Stone Age natural appetite has not adjusted to the world in which we now live is not a problem. They have changed their eating behaviour and decided, consciously or unconsciously, to restrain their natural appetite so that they do not eat whenever the opportunity presents itself. Many of them have realized that they look and feel better for not having regular second helpings. Or they have got the balance of their diets right, so that they enjoy plenty of foods, other than the high-fat and high-sugar foods that contribute most to weight problems.

Others, however, are, as some comedians might say, on a Seefood Diet – they see food and they eat it. And their problems are compounded because much of the readily available food in the developed world is non-nutritious 'junk' (i.e., fatty and sugary foods). Overeating these foods regularly in the context of a 'couch-potato, car-dependent' lifestyle, leads to being fat, and to other food-related health problems.

So, it is hardly surprising that we have become overweight (and sick) when our natural instincts, and 'society' at large, both conspire to undermine our best efforts not to put on weight. Just some of the influences that affect what we eat can be discovered in the following list of psychological, social and physiological factors:

• Do we know, or wish to accept, the connection between our food and our health?
• Do we have enough nutritional information available from food labels to enable us to make good food choices?
• Do we have enough money to spend on food: more importantly, do we spend it wisely?
• How much effort and/or thought are we prepared to put into feeding ourselves well?
• Are we being deliberately misled by food advertising?
• Do we have will-power to resist the machinations of food manu-facturers and supermarkets to make us spend more, often on non-nutritious foods?
• Is good, fresh, nutritious food available where we live, work and shop?
• Can we overcome, if necessary, familial, religious and cultural pressures to eat unsuitable food(s) or diets, or just too much food?
• Are we given the chance as babies, toddlers and children to develop healthy eating habits?
• Can women, in particular, resist the pressure to achieve unrealistic body images shown in women's magazines and other media?
• Are we able to deal with emotional difficulties (and other dis-satisfactions) in ways other than dieting or eating disorders?
• Is our hormonal and/or genetic make-up biased to leanness or weight problems?

And so on . . . and on . . . and on . . . for there are potentially as many food-related problems as there are people.

Genes and your appetite

Around 35 per cent of people with weight problems can thank their parents for their present difficulty. For that number of people have an inherited disposition to put on weight. The gene responsible for a high body mass index (the latest way of measuring whether you have a weight problem, page 43) has not yet been found. The suspicion is that it may not be a single major gene, but a major recessive gene with age-associated effects. Whatever the geneticists discover, around 35 per cent of obese children have two obese parents and the same number have normal-weight parents. The obese children of obese parents are getting heavier by about 10 BMI units (explanation of BMI, page 43) per generation and the prevalence of obesity is increasing from generation to generation in all the populations that have so far been studied. So, again, we face a growing problem.

One of the genetic traits that causes weight problems is linked to the way we burn up the calories we eat. Normal-weight people use 95–99 per cent of the energy from the food they eat for getting around and for body maintenance. But people with inherited weight problems may have a genetic tendency to lay down fat rather than build body protein. And, if they eat a lot of fatty foods, they will be even more prone to weight gain as fat is more readily stored by the body as fat.

It was previously thought that fat people had small appetites, and were victims of this situation. But it is now known that they burn up calories at the same rate as normal-weight people, but because they have more body cells they need more energy. In general they eat more high-calorie foods than lean people.

If their appetites were re-educated by following the advice in this book, for example, then

'. . . that, surfeiting, the Appetite may sicken, and so die'
    (*Twelfth Night*, I, i, 3).

Genes and the shape you are in

Where you store body fat, if you put on weight, is also an inherited trait in half the population. Waist to Hip Circumference Ratio (WHR) is the most popular measurement of fat distribution. A high WHR means that most of the fat is around the tummy and back area, making you apple-shaped (the fat deposit shape most likely to suffer heart disease). A low WHR means most of your fat collects around the hip and thighs making you pear-shaped.

No diet can target specific body areas such as the stomach, hips or thighs; it is not possible to spot-reduce through dieting. However, changes in dimensions can be achieved by a combination of diet and exercise - and exercise gives other benefits as well. But you cannot change your basic body shape.

Women tend to have more fat around their hips and thighs and therefore have a low WHR. Men are more likely to have a 'central' fat deposit around stomachs and backs which is one risk factor for heart disease (until after the menopause, when the protection afforded by hormones leaves women equally at risk of heart disease and other health problems).

It seems that the genes you inherit determine how likely you are to be constantly battling to prevent weight gain in specific body areas – or whether you enjoy a small amount of genetic protection from weight problems.

The good news is that, although you cannot choose your parents (and your genes), you can control your environment, which can either decrease or worsen the influence of your genes. In other words, the amount and type of food you eat, the amount of exercise you take, whether you smoke and/or drink, and so on, can either help you slim or result in even greater weight problems.

You can reduce fat deposits and alter your WHR. This is especially true of the fat around the tummy, which carries the greatest health risk. Fat in this area is the first to be used up when you diet and exercise more. The bad news for pear-shaped people who are unhappy with their shape is that they cannot alter their shape by losing weight, but they can become slimmer pear-shaped people.

However, the fact remains that the vast majority of people are overweight as a result of disturbances in their natural appetite, leading them to eat (or drink) more calories than they expend.

Adjusting your Natural Appetite

For a start, don't go on a diet – not in the conventional sense, anyway. Diets don't work.

During a diet, the metabolic rate undergoes a 'starvation response': it slows down so your body needs fewer calories to maintain the same weight. That's why, after an initial easy weight loss during the first two weeks – most of which is water and glycogen (energy stored in the liver for emergencies such as starvation) – weight loss becomes very difficult. Contrary to popular belief, combining diet with a lot of exercise might lead to even more extreme energy conservation by the body, making it even more difficult to lose weight.

Diets of 1,200 calories a day, and certainly no lower than 1,000 calories a day, help avoid detrimental changes in metabolism. Research shows that, if you diet at around 1,200 calories a day, you will lose weight slower than on a lower-calorie diet, but the lost weight will be far less likely to be regained.

Dieters who eat less than 1,000 calories a day lose too much lean muscle tissue. As good body shape – which is what most people diet for – depends on well-toned muscle or lean tissue, this is another argument against a low-calorie diet and for exercise which will determine good body shape.

The effect of dieting on fewer than 1,000 calories a day is for the body to hang on to fat to see it through the period of starvation. As women have a higher proportion of fat to muscle than men, any loss of lean tissue makes them look even fatter than before.

In addition, as you lose lean tissue the basal metabolic rate (the rate at which your resting body burns calories) goes down. So, a woman who has been consistently slimming on less than 1,000 calories a day will have to eat about 20 per cent less when she stops dieting.

One of the most convincing arguments against dieting below 1,000 calories a day is that you will put on weight after the diet while eating less than before. Chronic (or Yo-yo) dieters develop a higher percentage of body fat and slower metabolism, so that they find it increasingly difficult to lose weight.

Crash diets, especially very low-calorie diets of less than 600 calories a day based on meal replacements, which claim massive weight loss, encourage faddy eating and a cycle of starvation and bingeing that increases the risk of heart disease and the danger of death from arrhythmia (when the heartbeat is either too slow or too fast), should only be undertaken by people who are very overweight and only under medical supervision for short periods. There is a danger from these diets of losing too much muscle and also possibly protein from central organs, especially on some liquid diets that provide as little as 400 calories a day.

Even if meal replacement diets provide all the necessary vitamins and minerals in tablet form, they still have a devastating effect on the natural appetite cycle. People who use them are far more likely to regain the weight they have lost and become Yo-yo dieters, stuck in a repeated cycle of rapid weight loss and regain.

As a rule, when reducing the quantity of food, it is essential that the nutritional quality is high to avoid the danger of going short of essential nutrients (vitamins and minerals).

Restricting calorie intake too much will affect all body systems so that cells will not be generated to keep up with general body maintenance. Immunity, too, may suffer because vitamin and mineral intake will fall with a restricted diet and this will lower resistance, weakening immunity to disease and leaving the dieter tired and lethargic. And people in a depressed state are more likely to overeat.

Slimmer but dimmer

'. . . I have a woman's longing,
An appetite that I am sick withal'
  (*Troilus and Cressida*, III, iii, 237–8)

Dieting can also starve your brain. Studies on women slimmers show they have a reduced attention span, poor short-term memories and slow responses. The reason for reduced intellectual performance could be: anxiety about dieting and body shape occupying women's thoughts and so keeping their minds off the tasks in hand; reduced heart rate, implying lower arousal or alertness; the women could be continually distracted trying to suppress their natural appetite. Women whose natural appetite is in balance can eat what they want, when they want and be slimmer without being dimmer.

Adjusting your natural appetite

'As if increase of appetite had grown by what it fed on'
  (*Hamlet*, 1, ii, 144)

Adjusting your appetite through the natural diet and homeopathy is the key to solving weight problems, and more effective than going on a typical slimming diet.

A healthy well-functioning appetite works well because of three systems:

1 The physiological feedback (like a rumbling tummy) that triggers both hunger and satiety (a feeling of fullness when you have eaten enough). These are the signs of which you are aware.
2 The neurotransmitters that send messages to and from the brain about what and when you need to eat. We are unaware of these neurological events in our body.
3 The psychological feedback that controls your eating behaviour, which is influenced by your social situation and beliefs. We can control and influence these to a large extent.

The danger with dieting is that it desynchronizes the natural appetite system and results in erratic delivery of nutrients with abnormal triggering of physiological responses. In other words, the messages get out of synch. And our behaviour is no longer in line with our physiological needs. We eat when we don't need to and we put on weight. In some cases, treatment may be required by a health professional, but not before trying to get back in touch with your natural appetite.

Pills to switch appetite on and off

Scientists have now found the chemicals that the brain produces to switch the appetite on and off. The chemical that stops eating after a meal is probably produced in response to the intestine extending and/or a rise in blood-sugar level from food. Blocking production of the substance called GLP-1 (glucagon-like peptide 1) in rats caused them to double the amount they ate. Once researchers find exactly how the chemical works to regulate appetite and stop eating, drugs based on synthetic versions of the protein hormone could be taken as pills, or sniffed, by overweight people to stop them having second helpings or raiding the fridge.

The brain chemical that causes hunger pangs is called neuropeptide-Y. Scientists are working on producing a chemical to block production of the substance or switch off hunger sensations. Both drugs would be open to abuse, and would have to be taken under medical supervision.

Who knows what side-effects they would have, and whether they would cause irreversible disruption to the body's natural appetite mechanism? Far better to rebalance your natural appetite without recourse to drugs that will probably not be available for at least another twenty years.

What is your Natural Appetite?

'Swich appetit hath he to ete a mous'
(*The Maunciple's Tale*, Chaucer, 180)

When we talk about appetite (in relation to food) we are talking about hunger or a craving for food. But we also use appetite to describe a person's capacity for food: whether they are gourmands or gluttons, or, at the other extreme, the bird-like creatures who are so indifferent to food they just peck.

The second meaning is important because, today, when we eat three meals a day, we rarely experience appetite in the sense of real hunger. Our appetite or our desire to eat is more likely to be governed by our heads than our stomachs, and this is called mouth hunger.

Eating is, therefore, no longer fired by the basic instinct of appetite to secure the preservation of the individual (or the race or the gene), as it probably was from the Stone Age to relatively recent times.

Mouth hunger is what you experience when you think you are hungry and mouth food is what you snack on when you are not really hungry, but you are eating out of boredom, habit and an emotionally triggered need for 'comfort' food. Mouth hunger sends us scurrying to the fridge or biscuit tin when we are faced with an unpleasant task, or as a diversionary tactic from the tedium of work (such as during the ubiquitous tea break, when mouth hunger demands a biscuit).

However, mouth hunger does have a role. To be fair, it is also instinctive. It is designed to prevent our blood sugar plummeting so low that real (or stomach) hunger starts, making the stomach growl violently for food. But it can be a learned response to certain cues – such as the Pavlovian response (salivating for biscuits when making a pot of tea), or Winnie-the-Pooh's desire for 'a little something' at eleven each morning.

'I am weak with toil, yet strong in appetite'
   (*Cymbeline*, III, vi, 37)

Our other instincts can also prompt mouth hunger – for example, the sight and smell of a favourite food, like the aroma of freshly baked bread, piped around the supermarkets from in-store bakeries to stimulate our appetite for food so that we buy more than we need or want.

'. . . Epicurean cooks
Sharpen with cloyless sauce his appetite'
   (*Antony and Cleopatra*, II, i, 25)

Appetite in a wider sense can describe our drive to eat food in a lot of different situations. For example, after a large meal with a starter and a main course, which are savoury foods, you may still have an appetite for a sweet pudding, whereas if you were offered more savoury food, you might not eat another course. The body's natural appetite is for it to eat as many different foods as possible to widen the intake of different nutrients, such as vitamins and minerals.

Harmonizing your Natural Appetite

If your natural appetite is in balance, both forms of hunger (real and mouth) will work in harmony. The problem is that, today, we are often biochemically out of balance, so that mouth hunger predominates.

Brain chemicals such as serotonin, which stimulate the appetite, are hormone-like substances. Production is linked to the type of food eaten at the previous meal and the amount of exercise taken. The biggest danger is for sedentary people (most of us today) whose serotonin levels become raised, leading to a craving for mouth food. High serotonin levels are also linked with depression – and mouth food is eaten for comfort.

Food eaten as a result of mouth hunger can go on to stimulate the appetite even more, rather than satisfying it. The more tastes and textures that are experienced in the mouth during eating, the stronger the psychological and physiological messages that are sent back to the brain, saying the mouth is satisfied. However, many people, responding to cravings set off by mouth hunger, eat only one type of food, for example, burgers, or biscuits, or ice cream, or chocolate. Cravings also lead to food being gobbled down quickly. If food is not chewed well, the brain will receive the message to switch off mouth hunger more slowly, resulting in more calories being consumed.

One way round this is to eat foods that you experience a craving for very slowly and chew well. The theory is that by the fourth mouthful the taste buds will be sending messages to the brain that they are 'satisfied' with this food. Incidentally, satisfying a strong food craving promptly and moderately will also make the food craving go (if it doesn't, see Chapter 2, 'Balancing Your Diet with Homeopathy'). Continually denying yourself a food will intensify a craving until you risk an uncontrollable binge, as many 'chocoholics' know.

'. . . other women cloy
The appetites they feed, but she makes hungry
Where most she satisfies.'

   (*Antony and Cleopatra*, 11, ii, 236)

When the natural appetite is out of balance, a vicious circle may be set up. Appetite, as we have seen, is a complicated mechanism and works alongside taste. Whether we find a food appetizing or want to eat it depends to a large extent on how it tastes. Taste is one of the five senses that helps us evaluate our food: the other senses are smell, sight, touch and hearing.

When we are deciding whether or not we find a food appetizing, we are usually judging it by its appearance, flavour and texture. The fact that these senses work together is illustrated by experiments that show people give higher scores for flavour intensity to darker-coloured foods - even though they taste the same as paler versions (hence the food industry's enthusiasm for food colourings which can give poorer-quality foods 'visual flavour').

It is impossible to look at taste, or flavour, in isolation because flavour is a combination of taste and aroma; although temperature also influences the flavour. Ice-cream makers have to add a lot of 'flavour' because we get less taste from cold foods (and drinks). How we think a food tastes is also influenced by its texture, and in judging the texture, we are also using a combination of senses (vision and taste) to contribute to our conclusion.

There are four basic taste sensations: salt, sweet, sour and bitter – although you might consider metallic and astringency to be necessary additions to the list, and a taste called umami has been 'invented' to describe the sensation associated with the most ubiquitous of food flavour enhancers: monosodium glutamate (MSG or 621 – it has no E number).

We taste our food through taste buds. These are groups of cells that contain taste receptors located in papillae (special structures) on the tip, sides, rear and upper surfaces of the tongue. Sweetness is detected on the tip of the tongue, salt and sour on the sides and bitter at the rear of the tongue. Babies have around 10,000 taste buds in their mouth, with a concentration for sweet taste buds (the preferred taste) on the tip of the tongue. The number of taste buds diminishes to around 2,000 in adults (maybe why baby food tastes bland to adults). The loss of taste with ageing is compensated for by taste 'experience'. Try this . . . if you hold your nose and shut your eyes, you lose your sense of taste. You may think you are eating an avocado, for example, when you are eating a banana. The next time you have an injection at the dentist, try eating a yogurt before the effect of the anaesthetic has worn off. The yogurt will feel 'warm' and have no flavour on the half of your tongue that is still 'frozen', whereas the true flavour and temperature of the yogurt will register on the other side.

Experience also helps us work out when we have had enough to eat. As far as we are aware, there is no inbuilt mechanism in the mouth that signals when our total of food at a meal reaches, say, 500 calories, which is what we might expect to need. Although the mouth does give the brain positive feedback to carry on eating, if the experience is pleasant, the stomach and small intestine give negative feedback to stop eating.

In addition to learned experience, there are mechanisms that operate during and after meals to tell us when we have eaten enough, so that we do not overeat.

Different types of food have different effects. Starchy food results in strong, but short-lived signals to stop eating. It raises blood sugar quickly, so that we feel full quickly, but for a shorter time, although new studies suggest fat may not make us feel full for longer, as previously thought. However, fat takes a longer time to raise blood-sugar levels, so that a lot of high fat food can be eaten before satiety signals stop us eating. Because of their palatability, it is easy to over-eat fatty foods. Maybe, for this reason, we override our past experience and carry on eating, even though we know we have eaten too many calories.

Experiments show that we regulate the amount we eat on past experience. Where people have found about 500 calories to be a comfortable and satisfying amount to eat at a meal, scientists have altered the calorie content of that meal which seems to the eater to be the same food. It is only over time that the eater adjusts the amount they eat to compensate for changes in the calorie content of the meal.

This is good news – it means we can alter our learned responses to food and adjust what we eat and the amounts we eat to rebalance our natural appetite.

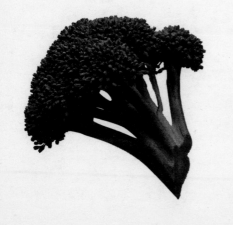

Chapter 2

Balancing Your Diet with Homeopathy

We have discussed what a natural appetite is and how, when our bodies are in physiological, neurological and psychological balance, we should be able, by listening to our natural appetite, to eat the foods we like in a sensible way, which will keep us at our proper weight and maintain health and vitality. We have also discussed some of the factors that lead us away from our natural appetite; these will be dealt with more fully in Chapter 5, 'Problem Solving'.

We have shown, however, that making contact with our natural appetite is dependent on external stress including social pressure, emotional stress, metabolic factors, genetic factors, physiological factors and so on. Despite this, most so-called weight-reduction diets are based purely on a list of foods that you should eat and shouldn't eat; whilst they pay lip service to the idea of other factors being involved, they are not taken into account as part of the general process of acquiring a natural appetite.

The origins for this go back to the medicalization of diet. Unfortunately, there is a split known as the Cartesian split in medicine, which separated the physical aspects of the body away from the more nebulous emotional and spiritual areas of our being. Thus, modern medicine has come more and more to rely on physical examination, investigation and treatment of illness, whilst largely ignoring the emotional and other areas, and psychological medicine tends to look at the workings of the mind, emotions and spirit, whilst neglecting the physical aspects. This is because the Cartesian model allows no room for a model of human beings that sees the mind and body as part of one being and not separated into two parts. This is about as logical as investigating the causes of road accidents by either examining the cars and ignoring the drivers, or looking at the drivers without taking into account the state of repair or performance of the car.

In order to fully integrate our model of how the natural appetite can be rediscovered, it is necessary to find a system of philosophy and therapeutics that has at its core a holistic model of health and disease. One of the systems of medicine that really fulfils this criterion is homeopathy. We will first look at the basic principles of homeopathy and then see how it can help us to get in touch with our natural appetite.

The History of Homeopathy

The ideas behind the principles of homeopathy date back to the fifth century BC, when Hippocrates (*c.* 470–400 BC) stated that illnesses could be cured by similars, by which he meant that, if a substance could be found which was capable of producing similar symptoms in a healthy person to those being suffered by the patient, then giving that substance to the patient would cure them. These ideas were not generally accepted.

It wasn't until the Middle Ages that Paracelsus (1493–1541) developed a similar philosophy which he called the Doctrine of Signatures, although here he meant that a disease can be treated by a plant or substance which had qualities similar to those of the diseased organ. For example, liver disease may be treated by greater celandine because it is yellow, and heart disease could be treated by plants that had heart-shaped leaves.

It wasn't, however, until the eighteenth century that Samuel Christian Hahnemann (1755–1843) formulated the laws of homeopathy as we know them today and homeopathy was really born.

Samuel Christian Hahnemann (1755–1843)

Hahnemann is recognized as the father of homeopathy. He was born in Dresden in 1755 and trained in languages, chemistry and medicine. After a brief career as a physician, during which time he was appalled by the medical practices of the day, he followed his conscience and left the medical profession to earn a living as a translator. Whilst he was translating a herbal book on materia medica by Dr Cullen of Edinburgh, he came across the statement that quinine was good for malaria because it was powerfully astringent – that is, it stopped the body becoming dehydrated. As a chemist, Hahnemann knew that there were many other substances and combinations of substances which were equally if not more powerfully astringent than quinine and he realized that there was something else about quinine that made it powerful in the treatment of malaria.

He performed an experiment on himself in which he took small doses of quinine for a few days. To his astonishment, he produced in himself the symptoms of malaria. He did not actually contract the disease or have a parasite in his bloodstream, but he did have many of the classical symptoms. When he stopped the quinine, the symptoms disappeared; when he started again, they reappeared. Just to be sure, he tried out the experiment on other people and found the same results. He then went on to 'prove' a number of substances and to obtain extremely detailed information about the effect that they could have in small doses.

He catalogued in fine detail the symptoms these substances could produce in terms of the physical, mental and emotional changes that people experienced. The next step was to start treating patients with illness with a remedy which was capable of producing similar symptoms in a healthy person to those that were being suffered by the patient who was ill. He found that the patients tended to get better, but he also noticed that they very often suffered from an initial aggravation of their symptoms. In an attempt to get over this, he began to dilute his medicines and he did this in a particular way. Not only did he dilute them, but he also shook them vigorously.

As he progressed in practice, he began to use higher and higher dilutions of medicine to a point where, according to physical science, it is very unlikely that even one molecule of the original substance exists. When he tried these new potentized medicines, as he called them, on patients, not only did he find that they suffered less aggravation but they tended to get better quickly – in other words, the medicines were more potent. This means the original substance from which the remedy has been made has been diluted and succussed 1:100 and repeated 30 times. This led him to formulate the two main laws of homeopathy.

The first one, known as the law of similars, states that a medicine can only completely cure a patient if it is capable of producing similar symptoms in a healthy person to those from which the patient is suffering. The second law states that the minimum dose is the one that should be used to effect this cure – in other words, the more highly diluted, potentized medicines work better than material ones. These two basic laws have stood the test of time, although they have been added to by subsequent generations of homeopaths. Being an essentially religious man, Hahnemann was intrigued to know upon what his remedies were working in order to effect a cure, because he was convinced that they were not working on a physical level. Being aware of the vitalistic theories of nature which abounded at the time, he reasoned that there existed within the body a subtle energy or Vital Force which not only gave life to human beings, but also was capable of curing them when they were injured or diseased. He felt most diseases occurred primarily in the Vital Force at first and that the symptoms of the illness were not due to the original cause of the disease, but rather to the body trying to heal the imbalance in the Vital Force. A rather crude analogy of this would be to say that the Vital Force is like a subtle master computer which sends out programs to run the tissues and organs of the body. If a glitch develops in the computer, the wrong program will be sent, as a result of which malfunctions will occur. Although it may be possible to modify the effects of these malfunctions, the only way to really cure it is to remove the glitch that caused the problem in the first place from the computer. Hahnemann's legacy to medicine, therefore, is not just a system of therapeutics, but a philosophical framework which enables us to see a patient not only as a physical entity, but also as a holistic being with a will, thoughts, feelings, dreams, aims and a purpose in life, all of which are completely part of that whole being.

The Spread of Homeopathy

In essence, what Hahnemann showed was that natural substances, some of which might be toxic to human beings, and others which might be inert, could be made to act on diseased human beings in a curative fashion if they were prescribed exactly according to the law of similars and particularly if they had been diluted and potentized by succussion. He saw that his remedies worked in a dynamic way – that is, they were not working on the substance of the body and its physical structure, but rather on the subtle or Vital Force in the body which not only gave it life but which was capable of healing its injuries and illnesses.

At the time he made these assertions, a growing number of physicians had become disillusioned with so-called allopathic medicine where most of the treatments were barbaric, to say the least, and more often than not caused more harm than good. Accordingly, during the nineteenth century, his ideas spread quickly from Germany across Europe and then to the Americas and Asia.

At the turn of the century in the United States of America, there were hundreds of homeopathic hospitals and over twenty university medical schools. By the end of the twenties, they had virtually been wiped out; the same would have happened in Britain if it had not been for the influence of the Royal Family and the aristocracy. In other parts of the world, however, homeopathy remained strong, particularly on the Indian sub-continent. The reason for the demise of homeopathy was partly to do with suspicion and greed amongst the practitioners of allopathic medicine, but perhaps, more importantly, because of a deep philosophical split within the ranks of homeopathy itself. This was between the so-called low-potency prescribers, who tended to view patients in a more materialistic way and to use low potencies of remedies, which acted mainly on the physical level, and the high-potency practitioners, who believed that most illness began in the mind and that therefore the whole constitution or essence of the patient should be treated, as well as the physical manifestations of the particular illness from which they suffered.

Since the 1960s, however, there has been an upsurge in homeopathy, much of it in reaction against the side effects of modern medicine and its lack of success, particularly with many chronic diseases. Today, homeopathy remains very popular in Asia and is growing in Europe and America. It is also strong in South America and growing rapidly in Australia, New Zealand and South Africa, but as yet has found little favour in Arabia and Japan. As it stands today, homeopathy represents a broad church, from doctors who use mainly combinations of low-potency medicines based on diagnosis, through to doctors and non-doctors who prescribe in classical high-potency holistic fashion.

Homeopathic medicines are also prescribed using techniques such as dowsing, vega machines and psionic medicine. These are not strictly homeopathic in the sense that they are not chosen by the law of similars. In many countries, low-potency homeopathic remedies are widely available over the counter in health food and chemist shops.

Homeopathy and a Natural Appetite

'. . . look you, this leek. Because, look you, you do not love it, nor your affections and your appetites and your disgestions doo's not agree with it . . .'
(*Henry V*, v, i, 22–4)

Homeopathy views human beings in a holistic way and it understands that any imbalance in human beings must ultimately be cured by human beings themselves. Medicines can help the body to heal itself, but every surgeon is well aware that, even though he can remove a diseased part from the body, it is up to the body then to heal the wound and repair the damage so that it can function again. When a homeopathic physician takes a history from a patient, he takes a very detailed look at the symptoms that the patient has, what makes the patient either better or worse; he also looks at the person who has got the disease or imbalance in their health in order to fully understand the whole picture of the disturbance.

Thus, in addition to the presenting complaint, he will also look at the type of foods that the patients like, dislike or get aggravation from; the sort of weather and environmental conditions that suit or do not suit them; how their memory, concentration and intellect work; how they are feeling emotionally, whether their will is strong and whether they have plenty of confidence in themselves. All of this builds up into a total picture that the homeopathic physician will then use to find a remedy which he knows can produce a similar picture in somebody who is healthy. When the correct remedy is given, very often the first sign that you will notice is a general improvement in well being, a feeling of inner strength and a strengthening of the will. This will then be followed some time later by improvement in the more physical aspects of the disease, so following the homeopathic law of cure that healing occurs from within outward and from above downward.

From what we have seen above, it is clear that a person's appetite and the foods that they like and dislike are not just some random fact that is set in stone, but are part of the whole picture of the person and irrevocably interwoven with their willpower, their intellectual ability, their emotional state and their physiological performance. Only when all of these factors are in harmony and balance can the natural appetite be experienced, leading to a balanced approach to eating, along with exercise and other measures. It is our belief that it is failure to understand this model of health and disease that has caused so many people to fail to achieve their ideal weight or to eat a balanced healthy diet. Indeed, most people know perfectly well what to eat and what not to eat in order to attain a satisfactory weight and healthy eating plan, and when they are honest they will tell us that they know what to do, but they lack the will-power to carry it out because of factor X or factor Y.

Often these factors are seen as external, such as the pressure of the job or children or marital problems, or that genetically and meta-bolically they are just built like that, or that they are addicted to a particular food and suffer withdrawal if they give it up. It is not, however, the external problems in life that screw us up, but rather our failure as human beings to overcome those problems. Psychothera-pists and counsellors have known this for a long time and many patients have been to them to try to deal with the underlying problems of lacking willpower. Many times the lack of willpower can be traced to feelings of low esteem and lack of self-confidence and discontentment, which often have their roots in childhood, school life and setbacks in life such as the death of a loved one, redundancy or divorce. Often, however, despite reaching an understanding of where these negative effects of the will arise, there seems to still be a failure to implement a proper programme of diet and exercise and other lifestyle modifications necessary to achieve a harmonious existence and a natural appetite.

This may be hard to understand but, still using the computer analogy: although the faulty programme has been identified, it is there because the original glitch remains and, because this is on a dynamic level, we believe that it can only be removed by a medicine which is capable of acting on the same level. Thus, we have found that homeopathy, by increasing the general well-being of the patient, frees the will to take on the challenge of finding the natural appetite. It may also be necessary for some counselling to help understand the nature of the bad habits that have led to the problem in the first place. Counselling and psychotherapy, however, on their own, may be unable to remove the causative fault and here homeopathy is an invaluable back-up system.

It will be obvious from everything we have said above that the more imbalances there are on the level of the will, the intellect and the emotions, or the more severe the physical symptoms are, the less suitable self-help measures will be. Thus, while we are attempting to give you an understanding of how you can use the principles and philosophy of homeopathy to gain an understanding of the new dimensions that you may need to look at in order to regain your natural appetite, it must be pointed out that it may not be possible for you to treat yourself and that you should seek the help of an experienced practitioner. In Chapter 6, 'Finding Your Homeopathic Food Type', we will be dealing with how you can treat yourself and when you should seek further help, and also how to take homeopathic medicines safely.

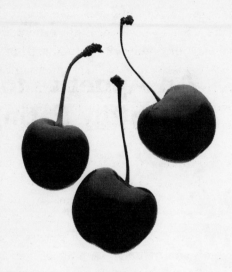

Chapter 3

An Appetite for Healthy Eating

Six thousand years ago when Stone Age hunter-gatherer man was armed only with a few stone instruments and a phylogenetic memory (for safe and dangerous plants), he was probably regularly eating between two hundred and three hundred different species of food.

Such a wide and varied diet provided a broad spectrum of fatty acids, vitamins and minerals and a huge array of secondary compounds (such as antioxidants, plant hormones, enzymes and other as yet undiscovered substances) that recent research suggests are vital for health. They probably act both alone and with vitamins and minerals – possibly in subtle, homeopathic ways – to promote health and protect us from disease.

Today, we are worse off for not eating such a wide diet as the hunter-gatherers, who had existed successfully on this planet until this century. A trip round the supermarket may be preferred by some people to foraging for corms, tubers and rhizomes in a wetland swamp, or fishing and hunting game in a marine estuary, but, for all its supposed 'choice', such a centralized system of food supply, and lack of biodiversity in agriculture, has reduced the variety of our diet to four or five staple food types.

Yet man remains an omnivore, able to eat a vast range of animal, vegetable and mineral foods. It is this diversity of food selection that has helped him evolve through thousands of years into the most 'successful' primate on Earth. Yet, ironically, we may be in more danger than our evolutionary predecessors of going short of the forty or so essential nutrients (fatty acids, vitamins and minerals) that have allowed our brain and nervous system to become far more developed than those of any other species.

While the omnivore's paradox (his ambivalence to new foods: wanting to try them coupled with caution) has helped man evolve, in other respects it has prevented him from reaching his potential. Man has always been hesitant, yet curious, to try new foods, with a 'taste-and-wait' approach. Once new foods had been tasted and no harm had resulted, they were perceived as familiar and acceptable, and were preferred above others. In recent times, this has led us to an even more limited diet, which relies on culinary skills to change the flavour and appearance of the same basic food types (e.g. wheat and meat) to stimulate the appetite, rather than eat from a wider variety of foods.

At the same time as we are limiting our intake of nutrients by eating a very limited variety of foods and risking undernutrition or malnutrition, we are also increasingly in danger of passive overconsumption (eating too much of these few foods) resulting in weight problems.

A further irony is that for all the so-called 'choice' offered by supermarkets and fast-food outlets, the quality of the food is such that we are unlikely to achieve our optimum health unless we have a finely tuned natural appetite and choose more wisely and widely.

Of more concern is the risk that we are not eating successfully enough to pass on healthy genes or maintain the intelligence of future generations at a time when we have social and medical conditions that allow us to survive into old age

Reverting to Your Natural Appetite

'. . . then to breakfast with
What appetite you have'
   (*Henry VIII*, III, ii, 203)

Breakfast like a king, dine like a prince and sup like a pauper, is the meal pattern that follows the body's natural appetite.

Breaking the night's fast with a substantial meal is how we used to eat when we rose with the lark and went to bed with the setting sun. In those days there was a good twelve-hour break between supper and breakfast, often with physical exercise before eating the first meal of the day, which certainly did build up an appetite for a hearty breakfast. And, when daylight hours were occupied with physical activities, you had the whole day to burn off the calories.

Reverting to this pattern, as closely as befits today's lifestyle, makes sense. If you eat well at breakfast, you still have the day ahead to burn off the calories. Eating a good lunch will avoid mid-afternoon attacks of the munchies and your head slumping onto your elbows for a snooze on the desk around 4 p.m. when blood sugar levels dip.

Avoiding heavy meals late at night makes sense because the digestive system wants to shut down for the night and you will get a better night's rest if you eat as early as possible – and that's not just advice for elderly people. It will benefit slimmers, too. After a night's sleep, the metabolic rate rises quickly to reach a peak at 10 a.m., where it stays through the day, until about 8 p.m., when it falls. Interestingly, most earlier cultures took the main meal of the day at around 10 a.m., a time that would now be considered a late breakfast. The second-best pattern is to eat small meals throughout the day (which need not lead to overeating) if your lifestyle forces you to eat your main meal at the end of the day.

'Sleep that knits up the ravell'd sleave of care,
The death of each day's life, sore labour's bath,
Balm of hurt minds, great Nature's second course,
Chief nourisher in life's feast.'
  (*Macbeth*, ii, ii, 36–9)

Whatever daily meal pattern suits your lifestyle, making a balanced choice of foods is about forming long-term healthy eating habits. Find your own happy medium to fit in with the custom and practice of your family and culture. Whether you eat two larger meals a day or six small/snack meals a day, ensure the overall content is well balanced – and does not exceed your calorie requirements. The most important thing is to make the balanced choice to meet your needs, ideally on a day-to-day basis, but certainly over a period of weeks.

'Or cloy the hungry edge of appetite
By bare imagination of a feast?'
  (*Richard II*, i, iii, 296–7)

Eating between meals is not a good idea, especially if you eat fatty and sugary foods such as sweets, chocolates, biscuits, crisps and cakes, because this reduces your appetite for more nutritious food such as vegetables, fruit, cereals and protein foods.

Of course, it won't kill you if you enjoy occasional meals that are high in fat and sugar. Problems arise when unbalanced choices regularly exclude more nutritious foods. Even then everyone varies and it is very difficult to say what the effects of any particular diet will have on an individual's health. However, it will be beneficial for everyone to make balanced choices from a variety of food groups.

What should we be eating?

One of the easiest ways to understand what constitutes healthy eating is to visualize a plate and think about the proportions of food from each of the four main food groups on that plate.

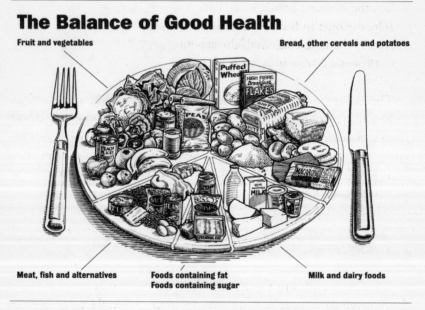

The Balance of Good Health

Fruit and vegetables

Bread, other cereals and potatoes

Meat, fish and alternatives

Foods containing fat
Foods containing sugar

Milk and dairy foods

(reproduced by permission of the Health Education Authority)

If you try to follow these proportions at most meals, then they will add up to the right balance of food.

The four main food groups are:

1 Bread, cereal and potato – 34 per cent of the food on your plate
Eat all types, and choose high fibre kinds whenever you can.
2 Vegetables and fruit – 33 per cent of the food on your plate
Choose a wide variety, especially those that are dark green and orange
coloured.
3 Milk and dairy foods – 15 per cent of the food on your plate
Choose lower-fat versions whenever you can.
4 Meat and alternatives – 12 per cent of the food on your plate
Choose lower-fat versions whenever you can.

Add an allowance of 7 per cent for 'extras' such as fats, and fatty and
sugary foods. Try not to eat them too often and have small amounts
when you do.

'. . . the sweetest honey
Is loathesome in his own deliciousness
And in the taste confounds the appetite.'
  (*Romeo and Juliet*, II, vi, 11–13)

The benefits of substituting artificial or intense sweeteners for sugar
or honey are dubious. Eating carbohydrate (starchy and sugary) foods
seems to naturally suppress appetite for more sweet foods; sweeteners do not seem to share this property, which can lead to over-
compensating for the calories that the sweetener did not contain.

'The fitchew nor the soiled horse goes to't
With a more riotous appetite.'
  (*King Lear*, IV, vi, 121–2)

While it is useful to think in terms of the approximate portions of
foods needed from each main food group, the Natural Diet recognizes
that everyone has different needs. The number of portions from each
food group suitable for you depends on many factors, including your
age, sex, how active you are and what your weight is.
  Only individual consultation with a dietitian, doctor or nurse will

provide a prescription of exactly how much you are likely to need from each food group. However, most people do not need this specialist advice, which is probably only necessary for Olympic athletes and others with very specific needs. But it *is* possible to work out more accurately what you should be putting on *your* plate.

What is a portion?

If, after seeing what frequency of portions is recommended for you (pp. 40–41), you do not want to increase the number of occasions on which you eat particular foods, remember the option of serving larger portions.

Bread, cereal and potatoes
Eat all types and choose high fibre whenever you can.

> 3tbsp of breakfast cereal
> 1 slice of bread or toast
> 1 bread roll, bap or bun
> 1 small pitta bread or chapatti
> 3 crackers or crispbreads
> 1 egg-sized potato
> 2tbsp rice, pasta or noodles (cooked)
> 2tbsp plantain, green banana or sweet potato (cooked)

Starchy carbohydrates are the best food source of energy. They also contain B vitamins for healthy nerves and digestion, and fibre for avoiding constipation and lowering blood cholesterol.

Vegetables and fruit
Choose a wide variety.

> 2tbsp of vegetables (cooked or raw) (see list on pp. 72–3)
> 1 small salad
> 1 piece of fresh fruit
> 2tbsp of stewed or canned fruit
> 1 small (100ml/3½ fl oz) fruit juice

Vegetables and fruits are the best source of: vitamin C for i_
and wound healing; carotenes for antioxidant protection agai_
disease and cancer; folates for prevention of anaemia and antic_
action (before and during pregnancy to prevent spina bifida);
and some starch.

Milk, cheese and yogurt
Choose low-fat alternatives.

⅓ pt/200ml full fat milk (gold, silver or red (homogenized) top)
⅓ pt/200ml semi-skimmed milk (red striped top)
⅓ pt/200ml skimmed milk (blue checked top)
1½oz/40g (matchbox-sized piece) cheddar-type cheese
Small pot (120g/4½oz) yogurt, cottage cheese, fromage frais

Dairy foods are the best source of calcium for strong bones, teeth and
nerves. They also provide some protein for growth and repair, vitamin
B12 to prevent anaemia, vitamins A and D for healthy eyes and bones,
and are especially important for babies and young children.

Meat, fish and alternatives
Choose lower-fat alternatives.

2–3oz/50–70g (size of pack of playing cards) beef, pork, ham,
lamb, liver, kidney, chicken, oily fish
4–5oz/100–150g white fish (not fried in batter)
3 fish fingers
2 eggs (up to 4 a week)
1½ oz/40g (matchbox-sized piece) cheddar-type cheese
3tbsp/200g/7oz baked beans or other cooked pulses, lentils, dhal
2tbsp/60g nuts, peanut butter or other nut products

These foods provide iron, which prevents anaemia, protein for growth
and repair, B vitamins for healthy nerves and digestion – especially
B12 for preventing anaemia – and the minerals zinc and magnesium
for growth, healthy skin and chemical reactions in the body.

Fats
Limit to 0–3 portions daily.

1tsp of margarine or butter
2tsp of low-fat spread
1tsp of vegetable oil (e.g. olive, sunflower, soy, corn, rapeseed).
Avoid lard, ghee and other hard fats
1tsp of mayonnaise, vinaigrette or other oily salad dressing

Fats supply mainly calories, plus some vitamin A and D needed particularly by babies and young children for growth. While vegetable fats also provide essential fatty acids and vitamin E, animal fats provide mainly saturated fat, so the nutrients they provide are better supplied by other foods.

Fatty and sugary foods
Limit to one per day.

Cream (and cream-based desserts and toppings), chocolate and chocolate spreads, crisps, biscuits, Danish pastries, doughnut, cake, ice-cream, jellies, rich sauces, fatty gravies, snack foods (such as Bombay mix and other savouries), soft drinks, sweets, sugar (in drinks, on cereals, in cakes, etc.), sugar confectionery, sausages and fatty bacon.

Fatty and sugary foods provide very few nutrients, but lots of fat, sugar and, sometimes, salt. The few vitamins and minerals they provide are supplied in larger quantities for fewer calories by foods in the four main food groups.

Composite foods

Beef stew, steak and kidney pudding, hot pot, Irish stew and so on are treated in the same way as fast foods such as pizza and other dishes like casseroles, lasagne and sandwiches, or 'ethnic' dishes such as bhajis, pakoras, speciality Chinese/Indian pastries, flans and quiches, moussaka and spaghetti bolognese.

You may be wondering how recipe dishes or foods such as pork pies fit into this way of composing a healthy diet. The way to deal with the foods listed is to identify the main food item or ingredient and then add other foods from different groups to build a balanced meal.

For example: a ham, cheese and mushroom pizza contains a dough base (from the bread, cereal and potatoes group); cheese (from the milk, cheese and yogurt group), ham (from the meat, fish and alternatives group). The proportion of vegetables, that is, mushroom and tomato relative to the other ingredients, is small, compared with the amount of vegetables and fruit on the plate. So add a mixed salad or cooked vegetables to the pizza, and eat a piece of fresh fruit for pudding to balance the meal.

Basing your diet on the proportions described above will satisfy the natural appetite for the pattern of eating that fuelled the evolution and development of the highly sophisticated brain and nervous system that differentiates man from other species. It will be a diet rich in the essential fatty acids, vitamins and minerals that are needed for optimum brain power, health and vitality.

The following suggested portions (*overleaf*) are for healthy people who are not overweight and not on a slimming diet.

Are you active or sedentary?

Exercise is vital for health, from building strong bones in childhood to preventing osteoporosis in old age; and it can do an enormous amount to improve body shape – the aim of most slimmers.

If you like sport or activities such as aerobics, between three and five 20-minute sessions of aerobic exercise a week can help you lose weight, lower your risk of heart disease, reduce stress and fatigue and improve flexibility.

Aerobic exercise means exercising to 60–80 per cent of your maximum heart rate. To discover your maximum heart rate, subtract your age in years from 220, which gives you the maximum heart rate in beats per minute for your aerobic sessions. Measure your heart rate

WOMEN

Number of portions

WOMEN	Bread, other cereals and potatoes	Vegetables and fruit	Milk and dairy foods	Meat, fish and alternatives	Fats	Fatty and sugary foods
11–14 ACTIVE	7–9 a day	at least five a day	3 a day	2–3 a day	0–3 a day	1 a day (if liked)
11–14 SEDENTARY	5–7 a day	at least five a day	2–3 a day	2–3 a day	0–3 a day	only occasionally
15–18 ACTIVE	9–11 a day	at least five a day	3 a day	3 a day	0–3 a day	1 a day (if liked)
15–18 SEDENTARY	6–8 a day	at least five a day	2–3 a day	2 a day	0–3 a day	only occasionally
19–49 ACTIVE	8–10 a day	at least five a day	3 a day	3 a day	0–3 a day	1 a day (if liked)
Pregnancy	one-tenth more from all food groups for the last three months					
Breast-feeding	a quarter more food from all the food groups					
19–49 SEDENTARY	6–8 a day	at least five a day	2–3 a day	2–3 a day	0–3 a day	only occasionally
50–65	6–8 a day	aim for five a day	2–3 a day	2 a day, choose oily fish	0–3 a day	only occasionally
65+	6–8 a day	aim for five a day	2–3 a day	2 a day, choose oily fish	0–3 a day	only occasionally

MEN

Number of portions

	Bread, other cereals and potatoes	Vegetables and fruit	Milk and dairy foods	Meat, fish and alternatives	Fats	Fatty and sugary foods
11–14 ACTIVE	9–11 day	at least five a day	3 a day	2–3 a day	0–3 a day	1–2 a day
11–14 SEDENTARY	7–9 a day	at least five a day	3 a day	2–3 a day	0–3 a day	1 a day
15–18 ACTIVE	10–14 a day	at least five a day	3 a day	3 a day	0–3 a day	1–2 a day
15–18 SEDENTARY	10–11 a day	at least five a day	3 a day	2–3 a day	0–3 a day	1–2 a day
19–49 ACTIVE	10–14 a day	at least five a day	3 a day	3 a day	0–3 a day	1–2 a day
19–49 SEDENTARY	10–11 a day	at least five a day	2–3 a day	2–3 a day	0–3 a day	1–2 a day
50–65	7–10 a day	at least five a day	2–3 a day	2–3 a day	0–3 a day	1 a day
65+	6–8 a day	at least five a day	2–3 a day	2–3 a day	0–3 a day	1 a day

by taking your pulse at your neck or wrist, and to start with, work to 50 per cent of your maximum capacity.

Target levels for different age groups

Age (men and women)	Target levels
16–34	Activity Level 5
35–54	Activity Level 4
55–74	Activity Level 3

Activity level scale

An Activity Level is of 20 minutes' duration in a four-week period. Different levels consist of varying numbers and combinations of moderate and vigorous activity.

5 Twelve or more occasions of vigorous activity
4 Twelve or more occasions of a mix of moderate and vigorous activity
3 Twelve or more occasions of moderate activity
2 Five to eleven occasions of a mix of moderate and vigorous activity
1 One to four occasions of a mix of moderate and vigorous activity

Moderate Activity

Long walks over two miles at a brisk or fast pace; football, swimming, tennis, aerobics and cycling if not out of breath or slightly sweaty, table tennis, golf, social dancing and exercises if it makes you out of breath or slightly sweaty, heavy DIY (mixing cement), heavy gardening (digging), heavy housework (spring cleaning).

Vigorous Activity

Hill walking at a brisk pace, squash, running, football, tennis, aerobics and cycling if it makes you out of breath or sweaty, some occupations that involve frequent climbing, lifting or carrying heavy loads.

If you have not exercised before, or are over thirty-five, check first with your family doctor, and have a proper fitness assessment and programme of suitable exercise worked out for you at a local authority class or private club.

Build up gradually to the targets above by first moving up from less strenuous activities until you reach or surpass your age target. Don't try to start at Activity Level 5.

Light Activity

Walking for two miles plus at an average or slow pace, light DIY such as decorating, table tennis, golf, social dancing and exercises that don't make you breathless or sweaty, bowls, fishing, darts and snooker.

However, if you do not like sport and do not want to take up a vigorous physical activity, then the Active for Life approach will suit you better. See page 145.

Are you the right weight?

Body Mass Index is a good indication of whether you are the correct weight.

To work out your BMI:

1 Measure your height in metres and multiply the figure by itself.
2 Measure your weight in kilograms.
3 Divide the weight by the height squared (i.e. the answer to question 1).

Check your result against the key below:

Category	BMI
underweight	less than 20
ideal	20–25
overweight; advisable to lose weight if you are under 50	25–30
you *should* lose weight	30–40
definitely too fat, lose weight now	greater than 40

Imperial height chart with approximate metric equivalents

4′ 10″	1.47m
4′ 11″	1.49m
5′	1.52m
5′ 1″	1.55m
5′ 2″	1.57m
5′ 3″	1.60m
5′ 4″	1.62m
5′ 5″	1.65m
5′ 6″	1.67m
5′ 7″	1.70m
5′ 8″	1.73m
5′ 9″	1.75m
5′ 10″	1.78m
5′ 11″	1.80m
6′	1.83m
6′ 1″	1.85m
6′ 2″	1.88m
6′ 3″	1.90m
6′ 4″	1.93m
6′ 5″	1.95m
6′ 6″	1.98m

How many calories in your food?

- Fat: 9 calories per gram
- Carbohydrates: 3.75 calories per gram
- Protein: 4 calories per gram
- Alcohol: 7 calories per gram

Your Natural Appetite for Fat

As we've seen previously, we have an inbuilt appetite for fat and fatty foods. As fats contain more calories than other foods, and seem to be laid down as body fat more readily than other foods, slimmers should limit their intake. In general, fats and fatty foods should not account for more than 30–35 per cent of calories.

Studies on men have shown that a diet containing as little as 20 per cent fat does not lead to negative energy balance in sedentary men. Moderately active men could eat 40 per cent of their diet in the form of fat and still be in slight negative energy balance (i.e., they could lose weight). This was not the case when 60 per cent of the diet was eaten as fats. From that it seems that there is a trade off between levels of physical activity and fat content of the diet. There may be a level at which dietary fat intake predisposes to weight gain as physical activity level decreases.

However, there are other good (health) reasons for limiting fat intake, too. Eating too much fat, and saturated fat in particular, increases the risk of heart disease by raising the level of harmful blood cholesterol. Cholesterol can build up in the arteries, slowing down the blood supply to the heart – or even cutting it off completely, causing a heart attack. Diets high in fat also increase the risk of some cancers.

Not all fats have the same effect. Saturated fats cause the most problems. Polyunsaturates are essential for health, and can help lower cholesterol levels. Monounsaturates share some of the benefits of polyunsaturates. All fats should be eaten in moderation.

Saturated fats

The ones we should be cutting down on are hard fats found in animal foods such as meat and dairy produce, hydrogenated vegetable fats and oils found mainly in hard and some soft margarine, cooking fats, cakes, biscuits, savoury snacks, chocolate and other processed foods. Too much of these is easily turned into unsightly 'storage' fat or 'spare tyres' (depending on where you are susceptible to weight gain, see page 7).

Polyunsaturated fats

There are two types of essential fatty acids which we need in limited amounts: linoleic and alpha-linolenic fatty acids are found in seed oils, e.g. sunflower, corn and soya oil, and dark green leaves and seeds. Omega-3 or similar derivatives are found in oily fish, e.g. mackerel, herring, sardines, tuna, pilchards, salmon. The body uses the two to build longer-chain fatty acids that make up the structure of the brain and nervous system. They are especially essential before and during pregnancy to ensure brain development and are a vital component of breast milk – 70 per cent of a newborn's energy from food and reserves is used by the brain for growth and maintenance.

Mono-unsaturated fats

Like other fats, too much is turned into body fat, and is found mainly in olive oil, groundnut and rapeseed oils, avocados, most nuts and some spreads.

A few dietary particulars

Butter or margarine?

Whichever you choose, use small amounts. Both contain the same number of calories and the same amount (80 per cent) of fat. What differentiates them is the type of fat they contain. Butter contains a higher proportion of saturated fat than soft spreading margarine. Hard block margarine is mainly saturated fat. A soft spreading margarine, or spread (e.g. Flora, which is 70 per cent fat), labelled 'high in polyunsaturates', is the best choice if you want to cut down on saturated fats. Or, use a margarine/spread that is high in monounsaturated fats.

If you want to cut calories and fat intake, choose a low-fat spread, preferably 'high in polyunsaturates' and with the lowest saturated and trans-fat content. A margarine/spread that is high in poly-/mono-unsaturates can also be used for baking. Alternatively, you might prefer a hard fat that is also labelled 'high in polyunsaturates'.

Low-fat spreads contain only 40 per cent fat, consequently they contain about half the calories. Reduced fat spreads vary in their fat content – check the nutritional label. Very low-fat spreads contain around 25 per cent fat. None of these products is suitable for cooking because of their high water content.

Which milk?

Full fat milk: 22g of fat per pint.
Semi-skimmed milk: 9g of fat per pint.
Skimmed milk: 0.6g of fat per pint.

If you have always used whole milk, semi-skimmed does not take much adjusting to because it tastes like whole milk. Skimmed milk has a much thinner taste and takes longer to get used to. Both contain as much calcium and protein as whole milk. If you really cannot get used to the taste of skimmed milk for use throughout the day, you could use it in cooking and drinks where the difference in flavour will be less noticeable.

What's wrong with sugar?

The popular myth is that sugar is good for you – especially if you are feeling tired. Lots of people think that sugar is a good provider of energy (calories). The reverse is true. It is a poor food, nutritionally speaking, because it provides only calories and no vitamins and minerals. It is also more likely to give you dental caries (holes in the teeth that need filling by the dentist) than naturally occurring sugars eaten as part of whole starchy foods, in fruit or in milk.

For these reasons it would be a good idea for most of us to halve our sugar consumption. This could also help with weight control. Sugar, confectionery, biscuit and cake manufacturers argue against the suggestion that sugary foods lead to weight problems. They say sugar as a form of calories is no more likely to make you fat than any other form of calories. While technically that may be true sugary foods (like fatty foods) are very palatable to many people, and it is easy to eat more (or too much) of a food you like. In addition, sugar does not contain any fibre to help you feel full up, so you eat more calories in a smaller amount of food – compare a popular chocolate bar with a couple of rounds of wholemeal salad sandwiches and you'll see what we mean.

In addition, eating sugary foods leaves less room in the diet for more nutritious foods. So cutting down on sugar (as well as fat) is logical, because it will reduce your calorie intake without decreasing your intake of essential vitamins and minerals.

Salty snacks

At the moment we eat about 13g (½oz) of sodium a day, which is equivalent to 2 ½tsp of salt. Only a fraction of that is needed and we would be better off eating far less. Aim for no more than 6g a day (1tsp) including the salt already present in prepared foods, especially as lowering sodium intake could be of benefit in reducing high blood pressure. In fact, you do not really need any added salt (unless you have special requirements) – there is enough naturally occurring sodium in the main food groups that make up the bulk of the diet.

Enough to drive you to drink?

The good news, for those who drink, is that so-called 'moderate drinking', which means one and a half to two drinks a day, has been associated with a longer, healthier life.

The best known example of this is the people of the Mediterranean, who drink wine as part of their traditional diet. The second point is important because a well-nourished body will cope better with alcohol.

So it might be necessary to add a rider and say that moderate drinking is OK, if it is part of a healthy diet and lifestyle (i.e. not smoking and taking enough exercise). As we have seen, the healthier diet is one rich in starchy foods, vegetables and fruit and low in fat.

While it would seem that you don't have to cut out alcohol, no health experts actually recommend alcohol because of the risk of adverse effects. The exception to any possible benefit is pregnant women (and women who think they may be pregnant or who are trying to become pregnant). No alcohol should be taken until the fourth month of pregnancy, when one or two drinks a week are 'allowed', but it is still best not to drink alcohol during pregnancy.

No disease has been associated with moderate levels of drinking, and moderate drinkers seem to be healthier than non-drinkers and heavy drinkers. Alcohol is still a substance that the body has to detoxify, a process that needs a good supply of vitamins C, B and some minerals – hence the need for a good diet.

Low-risk levels of alcohol were, until recently, 14 units a week for women and 21 for men. In December 1995, this advice was revised by the Department of Health – against the advice of doctors – because it was thought to be more helpful for people to think of a daily benchmark than a number of units per week. Revised advice is that one or two units a day gives health benefit in reducing heart disease for men over forty and post-menopausal women. While stating that men who drink three to four units a day and women who drink two to three units a day (women 14–21 a week, men 21–28) do not face a significant health risk, the DoH adds that consistently drinking that amount carries an increasing health risk! Pregnant women might also drink one or two units a week, says the new advice.

If you do drink, it is still considered unsafe to drink before or during driving, or when using machinery and electrical equipment. Spread alcoholic drinks throughout the week. Try to have some drink-free days in order to prevent alcohol becoming a habit. If you are overweight, remember that alcohol contains a lot of calories. Avoid getting drunk.

1 unit of alcohol = ½pt/300ml beer, lager
4½fl oz/120ml one small glass of wine
⅙ gill/25ml/1fl oz one pub measure of spirits

Do I need to give up meat?

Meat is widely eaten and enjoyed, and while it is not necessary to give it up, those who eat it should probably reduce the amount. Meat is a convenient form of protein, and we need to obtain essential amino acids that cannot be made in the body to build protein. But if your appetite is not for meat, there are plenty of other sources (see below) that can be equally satisfactory in a well-balanced diet, such as replacing some meat meals with fish or vegetarian alternatives.

Meat eaters have to be careful about the amount they eat because, while the right type of meat, i.e. lean, organic and free-range (not meat products like sausages, pies, pâtés, etc.), may be nutritious, meat contains a lot of fat, especially saturated fat. While the body can tolerate wide differences in diet, there are limits. Too much saturated fat results in atherosclerosis (hardened and narrowed arteries) and heart disease.

Organic and free-range meat (and other foods) have much to commend them, for both humanitarian and health reasons. Man's natural appetite for a mixed diet that includes meat and fish evolved when wild animals were far leaner and the fat they contained was far higher in essential polyunsaturated fats. For every 100 grams of fat/ lean meat derived from a factory farmed animal today we get 225 calories from the fat and 40 calories from the lean compared with a mere 36 per cent fat calories from a wild animal and 70 per cent lean. The carcase of domestic cattle that end up on our plates as meat today are 50 per cent lean meat compared with 75 per cent on wild animals and 25 per cent visible fat compared with 4 per cent in wild animals.

There are plenty of alternatives to meat: poultry, fish, eggs, nuts, beans and pulses, and new foods such as Quorn and soya-based products. These alternatives are all good sources of protein. Even cereals and vegetables contribute some protein; in Britain, we eat more protein than we need. In general, if you obtain enough calories, you will obtain enough protein.

Poultry is a good option for some main meals because it is lower in fat (served without skin). Poultry (and meat) produced from organic and *truly* free-range systems of farming contain even less fat; if the animals have led an active life (especially game), the meat will contain higher levels of polyunsaturated fats.

Fish is an excellent low-fat protein food. White fish (e.g. cod, haddock, plaice, whiting) is especially low in fat and rich in minerals. Oily fish (mackerel, salmon, sardines) is higher in fat, but the type of polyunsaturated fats it (and white fish) contains cannot be made in the body and are essential for health (especially brain and nervous system development); hence their name 'essential fatty acids'. They may also be protective against heart disease and cancer. In addition to minerals, oily fish also contains some vitamins.

Eggs are also nutritious and convenient food, especially free-range eggs for the humane and health reasons given above. However, caution is needed because there is still a risk of salmonella food poisoning from eggs that are not thoroughly cooked. Those at particular risk are babies and children, the elderly, pregnant women and anyone who is ill, for whom foods containing raw eggs (e.g. mayonnaise, some mousses/soufflés, egg-nog, some ice cream) or lightly cooked eggs (e.g. soufflés, scrambled eggs, omelette) are inadvisable.

Nuts and seeds are good sources of unsaturated fat (except for palm, macadamia and coconut), B vitamins for healthy nerves and digestion, some vitamin E (in nut oils) for reproduction and healthy heart, minerals such as iron to prevent anaemia, the antioxidant minerals copper, manganese and selenium and fibre. Nuts make a good alternative to meat, but they should be used in small quantities and as part of a main meal, not for snacks, because, although they are nutritious, they are very high in fat and, therefore, in calories.

Legumes (beans and pulses) are rich in protein (especially important in the vegetarian diet) for growth and repair, B vitamins for healthy nerves and digestion, fibre (unlike animal sources of protein) and minerals such as iron to prevent anaemia. The term also covers peas (including chickpeas) and lentils. They are fantastically versatile in cooking, cheap and have a wonderfully healthy eating profile, being low in fat, high in protein and fibre.

Vegetarians make better use of beans and lentils, and they should eat them on an almost daily basis to avoid being over-reliant on high fat dairy food for protein. Combined with cereals (bread and pasta) and grains (rice, etc.), beans provide the building blocks of protein in the right proportions.

Canned beans are very easy to use. They may be more expensive than cooking your own but they are still a lot cheaper than meat and other animal protein foods. When cooking your own beans from dried, soak well (according to pack or recipe instructions) before cooking, except for split red lentils. Ensure that the beans are boiled for at least ten minutes to destroy a substance that would otherwise lead to upset stomachs.

As beans and other pulses are used widely throughout the world, adding more recipes to your everyday food is an excellent way to enjoy new and exciting dishes and sample different cuisines from around the world.

Vegetarians and iron

The iron in meat is more easily used by the body. The same is true for zinc, another important mineral found in meat. Vegetarian sources of iron include whole grains, pulses, dried apricots and dark green vegetables. Eating or drinking vitamin C-rich foods and drinks at the same meal will help improve uptake of vegetarian iron.

For practical suggestions on food and cooking, plus recipes, see Chapter 4, 'The Natural Diet', and Chapter 7, 'The Natural Diet Maintenance Plan'.

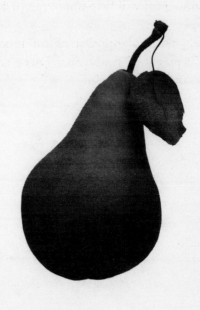

The Natural Diet

The natural appetite for slimmers

The basic version of the Natural Diet (in the left-hand column) is for women aged 19–50, who have a sedentary lifestyle, no health problems and want to lose weight. It is a rotating two-week diet based on 1,200 calories per day. It includes fish and poultry (game optional), but no red meat. There are Vegetarian options (*V*) in all the diets.

The Food Diary that accompanies the diet may be filled in on a daily basis. Note any food likes, dislikes and aggravations, plus food-related emotions that you experience before and while on the diet. The purpose of the diary is to obtain information which will help you to choose a homeopathic remedy to put your will, emotions, intellect and physiology into better balance and put you in touch with your natural appetite.

In addition to the basic Natural Diet of 1,200 calories for sedentary women, there are versions of the diet, which are given in the right-hand column where additions to the basic 1,200-calorie diet are listed, for active women, sedentary men and active men who also need to lose weight.

Substitute refers to specific items that replace those listed in the basic 1,200 calorie diet in the left-hand column.

The natural appetite for non-slimmers

If you do not want to lose weight, but would like to follow a healthy eating plan, then simply eat the same foods as for the groups above on their slimming diet, but in larger amounts. These have been worked out for the following groups who do not need to lose weight: non-slimming sedentary women, non-slimming active men, non-slimming sedentary men and non-slimming active women.

If you are pregnant, follow only non-slimming versions. If you have any medical condition that might preclude slimming, or if you experience side-effects on the diet, please consult your doctor (see also Chapter 5, 'Problem Solving').

General instructions

The diet is arranged over two weeks. Once you have completed week 1, you move on to week 2. During the third week, week 1 is repeated and during the fourth week, week 2 is repeated. However, if you prefer, you can repeat the first week for week 2 and use week 2's eating plan for weeks 3 and 4.

This is especially useful if you do not have a freezer, because some items are prepared in batches during weeks 1 and 3 and then frozen in readiness for weeks 2 and 4. Another option is to repeat the diet on a daily basis. For example, repeat each day's food twice – i.e. eat day 1's menu on days 1 and 2, day 2's menu on days 3 and 4. The latter arrangement has benefits when shopping for fresh foods. Whichever you choose, enjoy your food.

Shopping – weekly shopping lists are included. They allow you to take advantage of the 'batch' cooking. For example, in week 1, all the foods are listed for the main recipes that can be prepared in double portions and then frozen for week 3. The same applies for week 2, when foods may be prepared for week 4.

Drinks – some drinks are stipulated in the diet. In total, you need six to eight (non-alcoholic) drinks per day, but drink more if necessary (e.g. thirst, hot weather, sport). Water, diluted fruit juice and milk (if liked) are better than tea and coffee, which should be kept to a minimum (try herb or fruit teas instead). Avoid fizzy drinks, cola, sweetened fruit 'drinks'.

Organic – where possible, use organic foods and ingredients.

Bread – and breadcrumbs are wholemeal (or similar whole grain). Slices are medium thick from a large loaf. No spread on bread/toast, unless stated otherwise.

Sandwiches – two slices of bread are used, making two sandwiches.

Breakfast cereal – one average serving of no added sugar or low-sugar breakfast cereal (e.g. Shredded Wheat, Puffed Wheat, Cornflakes if not concerned about sodium, or no added sugar muesli = 40g, or two Weetabix).

Eggs – organic or free-range, size 3/medium.

Flour – wholemeal, or unbleached white.

Fruit juice – orange, apple, grapefruit, pineapple, unsweetened (1 glass = 125ml).

Margarine – high in polyunsaturates. If low fat spread is preferred, double the quantity may be used.

Milk – skimmed.

Preserves – no added sugar, jam or marmalade or fruit spread.

Vegetable oil – choose from: olive oil, sunflower, corn, soya, rapeseed.

Yogurt – very low fat, or low fat.

Recipes – most provide two portions. For explanation, see *Shopping lists*.

Shopping lists – reminder: Week 1 is repeated during week 3 and week 2 is repeated during week 4. You might, therefore, expect the shopping lists for both weeks 1 and 3 and weeks 2 and 4 to be the same. They are not. The ingredients for recipes which can be prepared in advance and frozen are listed in weeks 1 and 2. This means you can save time and effort by making double portions and freezing (or storing as appropriate) for when the dish appears again on the menu. But if you are not following the basic slimmers' diet, you may need to make double portions – check with the category you are following and adjust the amounts required on the basic shopping list *before* setting out for the shops.

DAYS	Breakfast	Lunch	Dinner
1 & 15	Fruit juice Muesli★ Toast	Egg sandwich Apple	Salmon steak, grilled V Sweetcorn polenta★ with Spicy Tomato sauce★ Fruit salad
2 & 16	Grapefruit Prunes Toast	Cheese and apple sandwich Yogurt	Chicken risotto★ V Vegetable risotto★ Baked apple with Date stuffing★
3 & 17	Fruit juice Porridge★	Tomato soup★ and Roll	Avocado and pasta salad★ Raisin pancake★
4 & 18	Fruit juice Breakfast cereal Banana	Tuna jacket potato★ V Cheese jacket potato★	Anchovy pasta★ V Spinach Gnocchi★ with tomato sauce★ Instant fruit fool★
5 & 19	Hot Cross bun Fruit compote	Cheese and carrot bap Yogurt	Haddock and prawn fishcake★ V Vegetable burger★ Blackberry and apple summer pudding★
6 & 20	Fruit juice Carrot and raisin muffin★	Hummus Toast Vegetables	Meatballs★ in tomato sauce V Nutballs★ Fruit yogurt
7 & 21	Fruit juice Carrot and raisin muffin★	Rollmops on rye V Carrot/Nut salad roll Yogurt	Roast chicken V Mediterranean Vegetable Pie★ Apple tart★

★Recipes given   V Vegetarian alternatives

DAYS	Breakfast	Lunch	Dinner
8 & 22	Fruit juice Porridge★	Pan bagna *V Veggie pan bagna*	Seafood lasagne★ *V Pepper and spinach* *lasagne★* Fruit kebabs
9 & 23	Grapefruit Prunes Toast	Tuna ciabatta *V Mozzarella* *Ciabatta* Yogurt	Chicken stir-fry★ *V Quorn stir-fry★* Sweet and sour sauce★ Fruit crunch★
10 & 24	Fruit juice Muesli Toast	Waldorf salad★ with yogurt dressing	Mackerel kebabs★ *V Nut shish kebabs★* Raisin pancake★
11 & 25	Fruit juice Breakfast cereal Banana	Turkey sandwich *V Bean tortilla with* *salsa*	Calzone/pizza turnover★ Coeur à la crème★ with fruit sauce
12 & 26	Hot Cross bun Fruit compote	Black bean and corn soup★ and roll	Fish steak, tortilla and salsa★ *V Rösti★* Trifle★
13 & 27	Fruit juice Savoury breakfast croissant★	Chicken and coleslaw sandwich *V Bruschetta★*	Salad niçoise *V Scotch egg★* Warm fruit brûlée★
14 & 28	Fruit juice Savoury breakfast croissant★	Goat's cheese and rocket salad	Rabbit/chicken casserole★ *V Minestrone casserole★* Orange and mango jelly

★Recipes given   *V Vegetarian alternatives*

59

Store cupboard/fridge items for entire (Basic) diet

Before you shop for the diet, check your store cupboard for the following items. Substitutes can be made – choose items for the same calorific value.

apricots, dried 175g
baking powder 3tsp
beans, black 75g
biscuits
    boudoir 4 or ratafia 8
    digestives 3
breadcrumbs (or flour) 15g
cereal, breakfast (e.g. Shredded Wheat, Puffed Wheat, Weetabix, no-added-sugar muesli, cornflakes) 4 servings
cornflour 2tsp (non-vegetarians +2tbsp)
dates 300g
flour, unbleached or wholemeal 740g (vegetarians +50g)
fruit salad, dried 450g
hazelnuts 70g (vegetarians +115g)
jam/marmalade 150g
jelly ½ packet
Jordans crunchy bar 1
lentils, split red 75g
margarine 170g (vegetarians +60g)
oats 450g
oil, olive/sunflower 135ml (vegetarians +45ml)
olives, black 18
passata 150ml
pasta of choice 150g fresh or 50g dry
    lasagne 75g
    penne, wholemeal 115g
pâté, fresh black olive 40g (or substitute Marmite)
pesto 40g (vegetarians +20g)
prunes, pitted 115g
raisins 140g
rice, brown 900g cooked weight, approx. 300g dry weight (including 115g arborio/risotto)
seeds, sunflower (or pine kernels) 40g

soy sauce 2tbsp
stock, vegetable 2.7 litres (vegetarians +450ml)
sugar (demerara/muscovado/fructose) 75g
syrup, organic maize malt (or honey) 200g
tomatoes
    canned 800g (vegetarians +400g)
    purée 40g (non-vegetarians +40g)
walnut pieces 50g
yeast 2 sachets or 25g fresh

Non-vegetarians
mustard 1tbsp
pine kernels 40g
vinegar 1tbsp

Vegetarians only
beans
    chilli (canned) 340g
    pinto (canned) 225g
cashews, chopped 115g

SPICES (GROUND)

cinnamon 1tsp
coriander 1tsp
cumin 1tsp
nutmeg ½tsp
turmeric ½tsp

Non-vegetarians
peppercorns 3
saffron, optional

Vegetarians only
garam masala 1tsp

HERBS

Non-vegetarians
bayleaf

Week I

Basic 1,200 calorie shopping list

VEGETABLES

avocado ½
broccoli 50g
carrots 5
celery sticks 1
courgette 2 (non-vegetarians +1)
garlic cloves 2 (vegetarians +1)
onions 2 (non-vegetarians +1½)
parsley, chopped 1tbsp
peas 115g
pepper, red 2½ (vegetarians +1)
potato 225g (non-vegetarians +400g)
   baking 1 (200g)
   new 175g
tomatoes, ripe 450g
watercress, bag/cress, punnet

Non-vegetarians
beetroot, baby 2
cabbage 1 portion
green salad leaves, mixed 1 portion

Vegetarians only
aubergine 1
beans, green 75g
chilli 1
corn, sweet 150g
pepper, green 1
spinach 115g

FRUIT

apples 6
bananas 1
blackberries 115g
grapefruit ½

grapes 8
orange 1
pear 1

HERBS

Non-vegetarians
parsley stalks

Vegetarians only
herbs, fresh mixed 2tsp
thyme, fresh 1tbsp
parsley to garnish

JUICE

apple 190ml
fruit 625ml

GROCERIES – frozen or chilled

filo pastry 1 pack
hummus 115g

Vegetarians only
polenta 75g
mushroom
   dried 20g or fresh 115g
tomato, sun-dried halves 6

DAIRY AND EGGS

eggs 3 (vegetarians +2)
cheese
   cheddar 75g (vegetarians +25g)
   low-fat soft 160g (non-vegetarians +75g)
   mozzarella, half-fat 1½ packs (125g)
   parmesan 2tbsp (vegetarians +2tbsp)
milk
   semi-skimmed 300ml
   skimmed 300ml (vegetarians +90ml)
yogurt 3 (vegetarians +1)
   natural 75g
   reduced fat Greek 75g

Vegetarians only
cottage cheese 50g

MEAT AND FISH (non-vegetarians)

anchovy 1 can (50g)
chicken, skinless 360g (additional 225g or rabbit/venison/pigeon)
haddock 175g
herring, rollmop 1
prawns, peeled 50g
salmon 150g
tuna in water 75g

BAKERY

bread
   12 slices wholemeal (non-vegetarians 2 slices rye or 14 wholemeal)
   rolls 2 (vegetarians +1)
wholemeal fruit bun 1

SNACKS (see p. 71 for list of snacks, p. 74 for symbols)

■ – 3 light
● – 2 light, 2 medium
  vegetarians – 3 light, 1 medium
▲ – 2 medium, 2 light
  vegetarians – 1 medium, 2 light
✚ – 4 medium, 1 light
  vegetarians – 5 medium, 1 light
◆ – 1 medium, 7 light
❑ – 4 medium, 3 light
  vegetarians – 5 medium, 4 light
○ – 5 medium, 5 light

Week 2

Basic 1,200 calorie shopping list

VEGETABLES

beans, french 50g
broccoli small head (non-vegetarians +50g)
carrots 1½ (vegetarians +1½)
celery sticks 1 (non-vegetarians +1)
chilli, red 1
corn, sweet 115g
garlic cloves 1 (non-vegetarians +1)
green salad leaves, mixed 1 portion
lettuce for pan bagna filling
mangetout 115g
mushrooms 50g (non-vegetarians +50g)
onions 2½ (non-vegetarians +½)
peas 2tbsp
pepper, red 3½ (vegetarians +1)
potato, new 50g (non-vegetarians +175g)
tomatoes 3 (non-vegetarians +1)
   plum 4 (vegetarians +2)

Non-vegetarians
cabbage, white for 1 portion coleslaw
chilli, red 1

Vegetarians only
courgette 1
leek ½
onion ½
pepper, yellow 1
potato, baking 1 (200g)
spinach 450g fresh/225g frozen
tomatoes, cherry 4

FRUIT

apple purée 115g
apples 1 (non-vegetarians +1)
blackberries, or other berries 225g
fruit
   free choice 1 piece

    free choice for trifle 115g
    seasonal for fruit kebabs
grapefruit ½
lemon juice, a squeeze
mango ½
oranges 2

Non-vegetarians
lime juice, a squeeze

HERBS

basil, fresh 15g pack (vegetarians 2 packs)
chopped fresh herbs of choice 1tsp
thyme ½tsp

Non-vegetarians
coriander, fresh ½ pack

Vegetarians only
parsley, chopped 1tbsp

JUICE

apple 150ml
fruit 625ml

DAIRY AND EGGS

buttermilk 150ml
cheese
    cheddar 25g (vegetarians +85g)
    goat's 60g (vegetarians +50g)
    mozzarella, half-fat 175g
    soft 165g (vegetarians +225g)
crème fraîche, half fat 100ml
custard, low fat 150ml/¼pt
eggs 1½ (vegetarians +1)
milk
    skimmed 300ml/½pt (non-vegetarians +300ml/½pt)
yogurt 1
    natural 2 tbsp
    reduced fat Greek 40g
    thick set natural/low-fat fromage frais 115g
    vanilla 1

Vegetarians only
cottage cheese 50g

MEAT AND FISH (non-vegetarians)

anchovy 1 can (50g)
chicken 300g
coley 115g
haddock, smoked 175g
mackerel 1
prawns, peeled 115g
rabbit or chicken 150g
swordfish/fresh tuna 150g
tuna in water 200g
turkey 50g

Vegetarian only
Quorn 350g/150g .

BAKERY

bread
    baguette ½ or french stick ¼
    2 slices (non-vegetarians +4)
    rolls 2
    ciabatta ¼ (vegetarian +¼)
    wholemeal fruit bun 1

Non-vegetarians
corn tortilla 2

Vegetarians only
breadcrumbs 15g
flour tortilla 1

SNACKS

■ – 2 light, 2 medium
● – 4 light
▲ – 3 medium, 2 light
✚ – 3 medium, 4 light
◆ – 6 medium, 4 light
❑ – 5 medium, 3 light
○ – 7 medium, 4 light

Week 3

Basic 1,200 calorie shopping list

VEGETABLES

avocado ½
carrots 2½
crudités, free choice 1 portion (e.g. celery, carrot, radicchio, cucumber,
    radish, pepper, etc.)
green vegetables, free choice 4 portions
peas 115g
potato 175g (non-vegetarians +115g)
    baking 1 (200g)
tomato 1
watercress, bag/cress, ½ punnet

Non-vegetarians
beetroot, baby 2
cabbage, 1 portion
courgette 2
green salad leaves, mixed 1 portion

FRUIT

apples 3
banana 1
grapefruit ½
grapes 8
orange 2
pear 1

JUICE

apple 165ml
fruit 500ml

GROCERIES

hummus 115g

DAIRY AND EGGS

cheese
    cheddar 50g (vegetarians +50g)
    mozzarella, half-fat ½ of 125g pack
    soft 40g (non-vegetarians +75g)
eggs 1
milk
    skimmed 300ml
yogurt 3 (vegetarians +1)
    natural 50g
    reduced fat Greek 50g

Vegetarians only
cottage cheese 50g

MEAT AND FISH (non-vegetarians)

chicken, skinless 150g
herring, rollmop 1
salmon 150g
tuna in water 75g

BAKERY

bread
    8 slices wholemeal (non-vegetarians +2 slices rye, or 10 slices
        wholemeal)
    rolls 2 (vegetarians 3)
    wholemeal fruit bun 1

SNACKS

■ – 3 light
● – 3 light, 2 medium
    vegetarians – 3 light, 1 medium
▲ – 2 medium, 2 light
    vegetarians – 1 medium, 2 light
✚ – 4 medium, 1 light
    vegetarians – 5 medium, 1 light
◆ – 1 medium, 7 light
❑ – 4 medium, 3 light
    vegetarians – 5 medium, 4 light
○ – 5 medium, 5 light

Week 4

Basic 1,200 calorie shopping list

VEGETABLES

broccoli 1 portion
carrots 1 (non-vegetarians +½)
celery sticks 1
chilli, red 1
garlic cloves 1
green salad leaves, mixed 1 portion
lettuce 1
onion 1
peas 1 portion
pepper, red 1 (vegetarians +1)
tomato 3 (non-vegetarians +1)
   plum 2

Non-vegetarians
cabbage, white for 1 portion coleslaw
chilli, red 1
potatoes, new 50g (non-vegetarians +175g)

Vegetarians only
leek ½
potato, medium 1
tomato, cherry 4

FRUIT

apple purée 115g
apples 1
blackberries, or other berries 225g
fruit
   free choice for trifle 115g
   seasonal for fruit kebabs
grapefruit ½
lemon juice, a squeeze
orange 2

Non-vegetarians
lime juice, a squeeze

HERBS

basil, fresh 15g pack

Non-vegetarians
coriander, fresh ½ pack

JUICE

apple 150ml
fruit 625ml

DAIRY AND EGGS

cheese
   goat's 60g (vegetarians +50g)
   soft 160g
crème fraîche, half fat 100ml
custard, low fat 150ml
eggs 2½
milk
   skimmed 300ml
yogurt 1
   natural 2tbsp
   reduced fat Greek 40g
   thick set natural/low-fat fromage frais 115g
   vanilla ½ pot

Vegetarians only
cheese
   cheddar 25g
   mozzarella, half fat 65g

MEAT AND FISH (non-vegetarians)

anchovy 1 can (50g)
coley 115g
mackerel 1
swordfish/fresh tuna 150g
tuna in water 200g
turkey 50g

BAKERY

bread
   baguette ½ or french stick ½
   2 slices (non-vegetarians +4)
   rolls 2

ciabatta ¼ (vegetarian +¼)
wholemeal fruit bun 1

Non-vegetarians
corn tortilla 1

Vegetarians only
breadcrumbs 15g
flour tortilla 1

SNACKS

■ – 2 light, 2 medium
● – 4 light
▲ – 3 medium, 2 light
✚ – 3 medium, 4 light
◆ – 6 medium, 4 light
❑ – 5 medium, 3 light
○ – 7 medium, 4 light

SNACKS

Light
fruit
vegetables
fruit or natural yogurt
plain currant bun
2 crisp rolls
large oatcake
4 crispbreads
1½ sweet biscuits
175g fresh fruit salad (no syrup)
175g canned fruit in juice
individual (around 120g) low-fat diet fruit yogurts and fromage frais
natural yogurt, low-fat 150g pots
frozen yogurt, up to two small scoops
low-calorie ice cream, usually called frozen dessert, 1 scoop
Ambrosia low-fat rice pudding, individual pot
jelly – any flavour, any amount!

Medium
wholemeal (fruit) scone
slice of malt loaf

wholemeal spiced/hot cross bun
300ml skimmed milk
small salads (without standard dressing), e.g. prawn, egg
small portion of stir-fry vegetables 200g
low-calorie sandwiches from supermarkets or Boots (around 200 calories)

Fruit – one piece unless stated otherwise
apple
apricots 4 fresh
½ avocado pear
banana (small)
berry fruits (raspberries, blackcurrants, gooseberries) and stewed fruit 4tbsp
clementine or other easy-peeling citrus fruit
dates 6 fresh or 4 dried
figs 5 fresh or 3 dried
grapefruit
grapes 115g
kiwifruit 2
mango ½
melon 175g
nectarine
passion fruit 5
pawpaw (papaya) ½
peach
pear
pineapple 115g
prunes 6 stewed or 4 semi-dried
watermelon 200g

Vegetables – portions of vegetables are 75–115g, unless stated otherwise
artichoke, globe
asparagus spears 5
baked beans (lentils, chickpeas, beans, etc.) 2tbsp
broad beans 2tbsp
french or runner beans
beansprouts (and other sprouted seeds) 8tbsp
broccoli and calabrese 2 medium spears
cabbage
carrots, sliced 2tbsp
cauliflower 8 florets
celery 3 sticks
coleslaw, low-fat 2 tbsp
cucumber 3-inch piece
leek

mushrooms, poached 12
mustard and cress ½ punnet
onion
parsnip
peas 3 tbsp
pepper
salad – green leaves, mixed
spinach
swede
sweetcorn 1 ear, corn on the cob
tomato 1 large or 6 cherry
turnip
watercress 1 bunch
yam (plantain)

Additional Food Allowances

Check to see which symbol applies to you, then look for it in the
Additional Foods column to find out what extra food you are allowed.

Calories
1450 Slimming active women ■
1550 slimming sedentary men ●
2000 slimming active men ▲
1900 non-slimming sedentary women ✚
2250 non-slimming active women ◆
2500 non-slimming sedentary men ❑
3000 non-slimming active men ○

Breakfast
Muesli 1 portion (see recipe)
1 glass fruit juice
1 slice toast spread with 10g margarine and
2tsp preserve

Lunch *Egg sandwich*
2 slices bread spread with 1 hard-boiled free-
range egg mashed with 1 tsp low-calorie
mayonnaise, pepper, unlimited chopped
watercress or cress. No spread.
1 apple

Dinner *Salmon steak and vegetables*
170g new potatoes
115g peas
1 courgette
150g Salmon steak, grilled (no added fat)
V Sweetcorn polenta with spicy tomato sauce
(see recipe)
1 portion green vegetables

Pudding *Fruit salad*
Make with washed but unpeeled ½ pear,
½ orange, 8 grapes, halved

ADDITIONAL FOODS

■ 1 portion muesli
1 slice bread/toast (no spread)

● ½ portion muesli
2 sandwiches
1 piece of fruit or 1 fruit juice

▲ 1 portion muesli
1 slice toast/spread/preserve
1 sandwich
SUBSTITUTE 225g salmon steak
1 piece of fruit or fruit juice

✚ 1 portion muesli
1 slice toast/spread/preserve
1 sandwich
½ portion potato
1 piece of fruit or fruit juice
1 light snack

◆ 1 portion muesli
1 slice toast/spread/preserve
1 slice bread (no spread)
1 sandwich
1 piece of fruit or fruit juice
2 light snacks

❑ Double portion muesli
1 extra toast/spread/preserve
2 rounds sandwiches
SUBSTITUTE 225g salmon steak
double portion potatoes
2 slices bread (with spread)
1 extra fruit juice
1 light snack

○ As for non-slimming sedentary man,
plus 225g jacket potato with 115g low-
fat soft cheese

FOOD DIARY

Strong Likes ....

Strong Dislikes ....

Aggravations ....

Emotions ....

Breakfast
½ grapefruit
4 prunes, stewed or ready to eat
1 slice toast spread with 10g margarine and
  2tsp preserve

Lunch *Cheese and apple sandwich*
2 slices bread spread with 40g low fat soft
  cheese and filled with ½ apple, chopped,
  ½ grated carrot and 20g grated cheddar
1 yogurt

Dinner *Chicken risotto* (see recipe)
V Vegetable Risotto (see recipe)

Pudding *Baked apple with date stuffing*
  (see recipe)

ADDITIONAL FOODS

■ 300ml skimmed milk
1 sandwich

● 2 sandwiches

▲ 1 slice toast/spread/preserve
2 sandwiches
1 portion risotto

✚ 300ml skimmed milk
2 sandwiches
½ portion risotto
1 medium snack

◆ 1 slice toast/spread/preserve
1 sandwich
1 portion risotto
1 medium snack
2 light snacks

❏ 1 slice toast/spread/preserve
2 sandwiches
2 portions risotto
1 medium snack

○ 300ml milk
1 slice toast/spread/preserve
2 sandwiches
2 portions risotto
2 baked apples
1 medium snack
1 light snack

FOOD DIARY

Strong Likes ....

Strong Dislikes ....

Aggravations ....

Emotions ....

Breakfast
1 glass fruit juice
Porridge (see recipe)

Lunch *Tomato soup* (see recipe)
1 wholemeal bread roll (no spread)

Dinner *Avocado and Pasta Salad* (see recipe)

Pudding *Raisin Pancake* (see recipe)
Makes 6, serve 1 with half a pot low-fat vanilla yogurt

ADDITIONAL FOODS

■ 1 portion soup
1 light snack

● 1 portion porridge
1 yogurt
1 light snack

▲ 1 portion porridge
1 yogurt
1 portion soup
½ portion Avocado and pasta salad
1 light snack

✚ 300ml skimmed milk
1 wholemeal roll
½ portion Avocado and pasta salad
1 pancake

◆ 1 portion porridge
1 wholemeal roll
1 yogurt
1 portion soup
½ portion Avocado and pasta salad
1 pancake
1 light snack

❏ 1 portion porridge
1 wholemeal roll
1 yogurt
1 portion soup
½ portion Avocado and pasta salad
1 pancake
1 slice toast/spread/preserve
1 medium snack
1 light snack

○ 1 portion porridge
1 slice toast/spread/preserve
1 portion soup
1 wholemeal roll
1 portion Avocado and pasta salad
1 pancake
1 yogurt
1 light snack

FOOD DIARY

Strong Likes ....

Strong Dislikes ....

Aggravations ....

Emotions ....

Breakfast
1 glass fruit juice
1 average 40g serving of no–added–sugar or low-sugar breakfast cereal, e.g. Shredded Wheat or Puffed Wheat or 2 Weetabix
150ml skimmed milk
1 small banana

Lunch *Tuna jacket potato* (see recipe)
V Cheese jacket potato (see recipe)

Dinner *Anchovy pasta* (see recipe)
V Spinach gnocchi with tomato sauce (see recipe)

Pudding *Instant fruit fool* (see recipe)

ADDITIONAL FOODS

■ 1 portion cereal/milk/banana

● 1 portion cereal/milk/banana
SUBSTITUTE 280g baked potato filled with 115g tuna in water and 75g low fat soft cheese
Vegetarian 250g baked potato filled with 40g grated cheddar

▲ 300ml skimmed milk
1 slice toast/spread/preserve
1 filled baked potato
½ portion Anchovy pasta/Spinach gnocchi

✚ 1 slice toast/spread/preserve
1 portion cereal/milk/banana
SUBSTITUTE 280g baked potato filled with 115g tuna in water and 75g low fat soft cheese

Vegetarian 225g baked potato filled with 40g grated cheddar
1 portion Instant fruit fool
1 medium snack

◆ 1 slice toast/spread/preserve
1 portion cereal/milk/banana
SUBSTITUTE 280g baked potato filled with 115g tuna in water and 75g low fat soft cheese
Vegetarian 250g baked potato filled with 40g grated cheddar
1 portion Anchovy pasta/Spinach gnocchi
1 large digestive biscuit (with the Instant fruit fool)
1 fruit juice
1 light snack

❑ 2 slices toast/spread/preserve
1 portion cereal/milk/banana
SUBSTITUTE 250g baked potato filled with 115g tuna in water and 75g low fat soft cheese
Vegetarian 250g baked potato filled with 40g grated cheddar
1 portion Anchovy pasta/Spinach gnocchi
2 large digestive biscuits (with the Instant fruit fool)
1 fruit juice

O 2 slices toast/spread/preserve
1 portion cereal/milk/banana
SUBSTITUTE 400g baked potato filled with 115g tuna in water and 75g low fat soft cheese
Vegetarian 400g baked potato filled with 50g grated cheddar
1 portion Anchovy pasta/Spinach gnocchi
2 large digestive biscuits (with the Instant fruit fool)
1 portion Instant fruit fool
1 fruit juice

FOOD DIARY

Strong Likes ....

Strong Dislikes ....

Aggravations ....

Emotions ....

Breakfast

1 wholemeal Hot Cross bun or similar spiced
fruit bun, toasted and spread with 10g
margarine

115g serving of fruit compote (dried fruit
stewed without sugar, e.g. prunes, apricots,
peaches, pears, apples)

Lunch

1 wholemeal roll filled with 25g low-fat soft
cheese, 25g cheddar, grated

1 small carrot, grated

½ punnet cress or watercress

1 yogurt

Dinner *Haddock and prawn fishcake* (see
recipe)

Serve 1 with 2 portions green vegetables of
choice

V Vegetable burger (see recipe)

Serve 1 with 2 portions green vegetables of
choice

Pudding *Blackberry and apple summer
pudding* (see recipe)

ADDITIONAL FOODS

■ 1 fishcake/vegetable burger
1 light snack

● 1 fishcake/vegetable burger
½ filled roll

▲ 1 filled roll
1 wholemeal bun and spread
1 fishcake/vegetable burger
1 light snack

✚ ½ filled roll
1 fishcake/vegetable burger
1 portion vegetables
1 medium snack

◆ 1 wholemeal Hot Cross bun/spread
1 filled roll
1 fishcake/vegetable burger
1 portion vegetables
1 light snack

❏ 1 wholemeal Hot Cross bun/spread
1 filled roll
1 fishcake/vegetable burger
1 portion vegetables
1 portion Blackberry and apple pudding
1 medium snack

○ 1 wholemeal Hot Cross bun/spread
1 portion fruit compote
1 filled roll
1 yogurt
2 fishcakes/vegetable burgers
1 portion vegetables
1 medium snack

FOOD DIARY

Strong Likes ....

Strong Dislikes ....

Aggravations ....

Emotions ....

Breakfast
1 glass fruit juice
Carrot and raisin muffin (see recipe)

Lunch
115g hummus
2 slices toast
unlimited raw vegetables, e.g. celery,
  radicchio, cucumber, carrot, radish,
  pepper

Dinner *Meatballs/Nutballs in tomato
  sauce* (see recipe)
Serve with 4tbsp boiled rice

Pudding
1 fruit yogurt

ADDITIONAL FOODS

■ 300ml skimmed milk
1 portion rice
1 light snack

● SUBSTITUTE 160g hummus
½ portion Meatballs/Nutballs in tomato
  sauce
1 light snack

▲ 1 muffin
SUBSTITUTE 160g hummus
1 portion Meatballs/Nutballs in tomato sauce
1 medium snack

✚ 300ml skimmed milk
1 muffin
SUBSTITUTE 160g hummus
1 slice bread/toast (no spread)
½ portion Meatballs/Nutballs in tomato
  sauce
1 medium snack

◆ 300ml skimmed milk
1 muffin
1 slice toast/spread/preserve
SUBSTITUTE 175g hummus
1 portion Meatballs/Nutballs in tomato sauce
1 slice toast (no spread)

❑ 300ml skimmed milk
1 portion cereal/milk/banana
SUBSTITUTE 175g hummus
1 slice bread/toast (no spread)
1 portion Meatballs/Nutballs in tomato sauce
1 medium snack
1 light snack

○ 300ml skimmed milk
1 portion cereal/milk/banana
SUBSTITUTE 175g hummus
2 portions Meatballs/Nutballs in tomato
  sauce
2 medium snacks
2 light snacks

FOOD DIARY

Strong Likes ....

Strong Dislikes ....

Aggravations ....

Emotions ....

Breakfast
1 glass fruit juice
Carrot and raisin muffin (see recipe)

Lunch
1 rollmop herring
2 baby beetroot
2 slices rye bread
mixed green salad (no dressing)
V Carrot/Nut salad roll
1 wholemeal roll split and spread with
  low fat spread and filled with ½ carrot,
  grated, 25g chopped cashew nuts, 50g
  cottage cheese
1 low fat yogurt (except **vegetarians**)

Dinner
150g roast chicken (no skin), low fat
  (thin) gravy, 115g boiled potatoes,
  unlimited carrots and cabbage
V Mediterranean vegetable pie (see
  recipe)

Pudding *Apple tart* (see recipe)

ADDITIONAL FOODS

■ 1 muffin
1 fruit juice
Vegetarian 1 muffin

● 1 muffin
1 fruit juice
1 medium snack
Vegetarian As above, except 1 light snack

▲ 1 muffin
1 portion roast chicken and vegetables
1 medium snack
Vegetarian 1 muffin
1 filled roll
1 yogurt
potatoes and vegetables with dinner as for
  non-vegetarian dinner

✚ 300ml skimmed milk
1 muffin
1 portion cereal/milk/banana
1 portion vegetables
Vegetarian 300ml skimmed milk
1 muffin
1 yogurt
potatoes and vegetables with dinner as for
  non-vegetarian dinner
1 fruit juice
1 medium snack

◆ 300ml skimmed milk
1 muffin
1 portion roast chicken and vegetables
1 portion cereal/milk/banana
Vegetarian 300ml skimmed milk
1 muffin
1 yogurt
potatoes and vegetables with dinner as for
  non-vegetarian dinner
1 fruit juice
1 filled roll
1 portion Apple tart

❑ 300ml skimmed milk
1 muffin
1 portion roast chicken/vegetables
1 portion cereal/milk/banana
1 fruit juice
1 medium snack
1 light snack

Vegetarian 300ml skimmed milk
1 muffin
1 portion cereal/milk/banana
1 yogurt
potatoes and vegetables with dinner as for
  non-vegetarian dinner
1 fruit juice
1 filled roll
1 portion Apple tart

O 300ml skimmed milk
1 muffin
1 portion cereal/milk/banana
1 rollmop
2 slices bread/spread
1 fruit juice
1 medium snack
1 light snack

Vegetarian 1 muffin
1 portion cereal/milk/banana
1 yogurt
potatoes and vegetables with dinner as for
  non-vegetarian dinner
1 fruit juice
1 filled roll
½ portion Mediterranean vegetable pie
1 portion Apple tart
1 piece of fruit
1 medium snack
1 light snack

FOOD DIARY

Strong Likes ....

Strong Dislikes ....

Aggravations ....

Emotions ....

Breakfast
1 glass fruit juice
Porridge (see recipe)

Lunch *Pan bagna*
¼ French stick or ½ baguette spread with
  25g black olive pâté and filled with 1 hard-
  boiled egg, unlimited tomato, pepper,
  onion, lettuce and 25g anchovies, drained
  on absorbent kitchen paper
V Veggie pan bagna
Omit anchovies and add 50g grated cheddar

Dinner *Seafood Lasagne* (see recipe)
V Pepper and spinach lasagne (see recipe)

Pudding *Fruit kebabs*
Arrange seasonal fruit on wooden kebab or
  satay skewers. Cut into bite-size pieces, if
  necessary

ADDITIONAL FOODS

■ 1 yogurt
½ Pan bagna

● 300ml skimmed milk
½ Pan bagna
1 light snack

▲ 300ml skimmed milk
1 slice toast/spread/preserve
1 Pan bagna
1 piece fruit
1 medium snack

✦ 300ml skimmed milk
1 slice toast/spread/preserve
½ Pan bagna
1 piece fruit
1 medium snack
1 light snack

◆ 300ml skimmed milk
1 slice toast/spread/preserve
½ Pan bagna
1 piece fruit
1 yogurt
½ portion lasagne
1 medium snack
2 light snacks

❑ 300ml skimmed milk
1 portion porridge
1 Pan bagna
1 yogurt
½ portion lasagne
1 fruit kebab
1 light snack

○ 1 fruit juice
300ml skimmed milk
1 portion porridge
1 slice toast/spread/preserve
1 Pan bagna
1 portion lasagne
1 fruit kebab
1 medium snack
1 light snack

FOOD DIARY

Strong Likes ....

Strong Dislikes ....

Aggravations ....

Emotions ....

Breakfast

½ grapefruit

4 prunes, stewed or ready to eat, served with half a pot of low-fat vanilla yogurt

1 slice toast spread with 10g margarine and 2tsp preserve

Lunch *Tuna ciabatta*

¼ ciabatta loaf (no spread) cut in half and filled with 115g tuna in water, drained, unlimited tomato and lettuce

V Mozzarella ciabatta

¼ ciabatta loaf (no spread) cut in half and filled with 65g half-fat mozzarella, unlimited tomato, black olives and fresh chopped basil

1 yogurt

Dinner *Chicken stir-fry* (see recipe)
V Quorn stir-fry (see recipe)

Pudding *Fruit crunch* (see recipe)

ADDITIONAL FOODS

■ ½ portion stir-fry
1 medium snack

● 1 portion stir-fry
1 light snack

▲ 2 slices toast/spread/preserve
1 ciabatta
1 portion stir-fry

✚ 1 ciabatta
½ portion stir-fry
½ portion Fruit crunch
1 medium snack

◆ 300ml skimmed milk
1 slice toast/spread/preserve
1 ciabatta
1 stir-fry
1 light snack

❑ 300ml skimmed milk
1 slice toast/spread/preserve
1 ciabatta
1 portion stir-fry
25g (dry weight) rice
½ portion Fruit crunch
1 medium snack
1 light snack

○ 600ml skimmed milk
1 slice toast/spread/preserve
1 ciabatta
1 portion stir-fry
50g (dry weight) rice
1 portion Fruit crunch
2 medium snacks

FOOD DIARY

Strong Likes ....

Strong Dislikes ....

Aggravations ....

Emotions ....

Breakfast
1 glass fruit juice
Muesli 1 portion (see recipe)
1 slice toast spread with 10g margarine and
  2tsp preserve

Lunch *Waldorf Salad* (see recipe)
Yogurt dressing (see recipe)
1 wholemeal roll

Dinner *2 Mackerel Kebabs* (see recipe)
2 Nut Shish Kebabs (see recipe for Nutballs,
  day 6) served with 4 tbsp cooked rice, 1
  portion each of peas and broccoli

Pudding *Raisin pancake* (see recipe)

ADDITIONAL FOODS

■ 1 portion muesli

● 1 portion Waldorf salad/dressing
1 wholemeal roll

▲ 1 portion Waldorf salad/dressing
1 wholemeal roll
2 Kebabs
1 portion rice

✚ 1 portion muesli
300ml skimmed milk
1 portion Waldorf salad
1 wholemeal roll

◆ 1 portion muesli
300ml skimmed milk
1 portion Waldorf salad
1 wholemeal roll
1 Kebab
1 portion rice
2 medium snacks

❑ 1 portion muesli
300ml skimmed milk
1 slice toast/spread/preserve
1 portion Waldorf salad
1 wholemeal roll
2 kebabs
1 portion rice
1 portion vegetables
1 Raisin pancake

○ 1 portion muesli
300ml skimmed milk
1 portion Waldorf salad
1 wholemeal roll
2 kebabs
2 portions rice
1 portion vegetables
1 Raisin pancake
200g jacket potato
225g baked beans

FOOD DIARY

Strong Likes ....

Strong Dislikes ....

Aggravations ....

Emotions ....

Breakfast

1 glass fruit juice
1 average 40g serving of no-added-sugar or low-sugar breakfast cereal, e.g. Shredded Wheat or Puffed Wheat or 2 Weetabix
150ml skimmed milk
1 small banana

Lunch *Turkey sandwich*

2 slices bread spread with 10g margarine filled with 50g turkey (no skin) and 1 tomato, sliced

Vegetarian Bean Tortilla

1 flour tortilla filled with 175g canned or cooked chilli beans, unlimited lettuce, tomato, pepper and tomato. Serve with 1 portion *Salsa* (see recipe)
1 piece fruit

Dinner *Calzone (pizza turnover)* (see recipe)

Pudding *Coeur à la Crème* (see recipe)

ADDITIONAL FOODS

■ 300ml skimmed milk
1 sandwich/½ tortilla

● ½ Calzone
1 portion green or mixed salad
1 portion of Yogurt dressing (see recipe)
1 light snack

▲ 300ml skimmed milk
1 slice toast/spread/preserve
2 sandwiches/1 tortilla
½ Calzone

✚ 300ml skimmed milk
1 slice toast/spread/preserve
1 sandwich/½ tortilla
½ Calzone
1 portion green or mixed salad
1 portion of Yogurt dressing (see recipe)
1 light snack

◆ 300ml skimmed milk
1 slice toast/spread/preserve
2 sandwiches/1 tortilla
½ Calzone
1 portion green or mixed salad
1 portion of Yogurt dressing (see recipe)
1 medium snack

❑ 300ml skimmed milk
1 slice toast/spread/preserve
2 sandwiches/½ tortilla
½ Calzone
1 portion green or mixed salad with 1 portion Yogurt dressing (see recipe)
2 medium snacks

○ 300ml skimmed milk
1 slice toast/spread/preserve
1 portion cereal/milk/½ banana
2 sandwiches/1 tortilla
1½ Calzone
1 portion green or mixed salad
1 portion of Yogurt dressing (see recipe)
1 light snack

FOOD DIARY

Strong Likes ....

Strong Dislikes ....

Aggravations ....

Emotions ....

Breakfast
1 wholemeal Hot Cross bun or similar spiced fruit bun, toasted and spread with 10g margarine

115g serving of fruit compote (dried fruit stewed without sugar, e.g. prunes, apricots, peaches, pears, apples)

Lunch Black bean and corn soup (see recipe)
1 wholemeal roll

Dinner Fish steak, tortilla and salsa
150g steak of tuna or swordfish

1 corn tortilla (Mexican pancake)

1 portion salsa (see recipe for day 11)

Grill the fish steak for about 7 minutes each side (depending on thickness) without added fat. To warm tortilla, wrap in microwavable film or paper or a wet cloth napkin and microwave according to pack instructions. Alternatively heat for 20 seconds each side in a heavy-based dry frying pan.

V Rösti (see recipe)

Mixed green salad (no dressing)

Pudding Trifle (see recipe)

ADDITIONAL FOODS

■ 300ml skimmed milk
1 tortilla
1 portion green vegetables
1 piece fruit

● 300ml skimmed milk
½ Hot Cross bun
1 portion green vegetables
1 piece fruit

▲ 300ml skimmed milk
1 Hot Cross bun
1 portion soup
1 roll
1 portion green vegetables
2 tortillas

✚ 300ml skimmed milk
1 Hot Cross bun
1 portion soup
1 portion green vegetables
2 tortillas
1 light snack

◆ 300ml skimmed milk

❑ 600ml skimmed milk
1 Hot Cross bun/spread
1 portion soup
1 wholemeal roll
SUBSTITUTE 200g fish/1 ½ Rösti
1 portion green vegetables
2 tortillas
1 yogurt
½ portion Trifle

○ 600ml skimmed milk
1 Hot Cross bun/spread
1 portion soup
1 wholemeal roll
SUBSTITUTE 225g fish/1 ½ Rösti
1 portion green vegetables
3 tortillas
1 yogurt
2 portions Trifle
2 medium snacks
1 light snack (2 for vegetarians)
1 piece fruit

FOOD DIARY

Strong Likes ....

Strong Dislikes ....

Aggravations ....

Emotions ....

Breakfast
1 glass fruit juice
1 *Savoury breakfast croissant* (see recipe)

Lunch *Chicken and Coleslaw Sandwich*
2 slices bread
½ carrot
shredded white cabbage
1tbsp reduced fat mayonnaise
60g chicken (no skin)
V Bruschetta (see recipe)
Mixed green salad (no dressing)

Dinner *Salad niçoise*
Arrange the following ingredients on a bed
  of shredded lettuce: 175g cold new
  potatoes, 1 hard-boiled egg, 1 tomato,
  sliced, 50g French beans, 25g anchovies,
  drained, 75g tuna canned in water, drained,
  6 black olives
Dressing: 1tbsp olive oil, ½tsp vinegar,
  ½tsp mustard
V Scotch egg (see recipe)

Pudding *Warm fruit brûlée* (see recipe)

ADDITIONAL FOODS

■ 300ml skimmed milk
1 portion brûlée
1 light snack

● 2 sandwiches/1 bruschetta

▲ 300ml skimmed milk
2 sandwiches/1 bruschetta
½ portion brûlée
½ portion Salad niçoise/Scotch egg
1 light snack

✚ 300ml skimmed milk
1 sandwich/½ bruschetta
½ portion Salad niçoise/Scotch egg
1 portion brûlée
1 medium snack

◆ 300ml skimmed milk
1 portion cereal/milk/½ banana
2 sandwiches/1 bruschetta
½ portion Salad niçoise/Scotch egg
1 portion brûlée
1 light snack

❑ 300ml skimmed milk
1 croissant
1 portion cereal/milk/½ banana
2 sandwiches/1 bruschetta
½ portion Salad niçoise/Scotch egg
1 portion brûlée
1 medium snack

O 300ml skimmed milk
1 croissant
1 portion cereal/milk/½ banana
2 sandwiches/1 bruschetta
½ portion Salad niçoise
1 portion brûlée
1 yogurt
2 slices of bread/spread
1 medium snack

FOOD DIARY

Strong Likes ....

Strong Dislikes ....

Aggravations ....

Emotions ....

Breakfast
1 glass fruit juice
1 Savoury breakfast croissant (see recipe)

Lunch *Goat's cheese and rocket salad*
Toast one side of 2–3 slices of French stick (or Granary/wholemeal stick). Top the toast with 60g goat's cheese. Serve with unlimited green salad using peppery hot leaves, e.g. rocket, watercress, radish and tomato.

Dinner *Rabbit/chicken casserole* (see recipe)
V Minestrone casserole with Pesto sauce (see recipe)
Brown rice, boiled

Pudding *Orange and mango jelly*

ADDITIONAL FOODS

■ 300ml skimmed milk
1 medium snack
1 light snack

● 300ml skimmed milk
1 croissant
1 light snack

▲ 300ml skimmed milk
1 portion cereal/milk/banana
1 bread roll
½ portion casserole
1 medium snack
1 light snack

✦ 300ml skimmed milk
1 portion cereal/milk/banana
1 bread roll
½ portion casserole
1 light snack

◆ 300ml skimmed milk
1 portion cereal/milk/banana
1 bread roll
1 portion casserole
2 portions green vegetables/**vegetarian:** large green salad with Yogurt dressing (see recipe)
1 medium snack

❑ 300ml skimmed milk
1 portion cereal/milk/banana
1 croissant
1 bread roll
1 portion casserole
2 portions green vegetables/**vegetarian:** large green salad with Yogurt dressing (see recipe)
1 medium snack
1 light snack

○ 300ml skimmed milk
1 portion cereal/milk/banana
1 croissant
1 bread roll
1 portion casserole
2 portions green vegetables/**vegetarian:** large green salad with Yogurt dressing (see recipe)
1 medium snack
1 light snack
225g jacket potato with 115g low-fat soft cheese

FOOD DIARY

Strong Likes ....

Strong Dislikes ....

Aggravations ....

Emotions ....

Eating out with the Natural Diet

If eating out is the norm for you, rather than the exception, or if you are unable to prepare your own meals, or buy your own food, thus making it impossible to follow the Natural Diet, use the following tips to make the best choices from the foods available to you.

Although you are not following the diet, you can still fill in the Food Diary to discover your homeopathic food type and rebalance any cravings or other disorders that impede you following a healthy diet.

Remember, these 'rules' apply to people eating out on a very regular basis. They are not killjoy rules, precluding the occasional treat when you may enjoy rich foods (if you like them) without ruining your generally healthy eating habits. The tips below are to prevent treats becoming habits for the 'business person', since it is long-term eating patterns that will really make the difference to your health and fitness.

Aperitifs

Avoid alcohol to save you 'empty' (i.e. non-nutritional) calories. Fruit juices are a better choice. *Choose* mineral water as a 'sociably acceptable' alternative.
Avoid crisps, peanuts and other salty/fatty savoury snacks, dips. *Choose* grissini (breadsticks) or bread (whether you butter it is up to you).

Starters

Avoid pâtés and meat/fish mousses. *Choose* smoked fish or gravad lax.
Avoid fried foods, such as goujons of fish or whitebait, especially if they come with creamy or mayonnaise (tartare) sauces.
Avoid salads served ready dressed. *Choose* salads with the dressing on the side, or stipulate no dressing in the preparation.
Avoid cream of, or creamed, soups. *Choose* clear soups, consommés, bouillons or broths.

Main course

Avoid fish in batter. *Choose* fish that is grilled (except meunière), poached or steamed.
Avoid meat in cream and other rich sauces. *Choose* lean meat, grilled or roasted, and remove visible fat.
Avoid fatty meat such as duck or roast lamb. *Choose* leaner game, poultry or fish.

Cheese course

In France, you might find a lowish calorie fresh cheese to eat with berries, instead of a pudding. In general, avoid this course entirely (unless you have not had a starter and you are not having a pudding). If you can't resist, choose cheese, but do not butter accompanying biscuits/bread. Better to accompany cheese with fruit or celery and eat only small portions.

Pudding/dessert

Avoid entirely, on a regular basis, especially if you have already had two courses. Starter and main course are usually of better nutritional value than a pudding – unless it's fruit
Avoid, in particular, pastries, soufflés, mousses, gâteaus, crème caramels, bread and butter puddings, pies or cheesecakes. *Choose* fruit, fruit salad or sorbet.

Coffee

Avoid cappuccino, Irish coffee and coffee with liqueurs. *Choose* black coffee or herb/fruit tea.

Petits fours, Liqueurs

Avoid these and the after-dinner mints and chocolates.

	BREAKFAST	LUNCH	DINNER
Days 1 & 15	*Fruit juice*: make sure it's unsweetened, or, better still freshly pressed. *Muesli*: skip the Alpen (or other sugary muesli) and choose a lower sugar cereal. Ask for skimmed milk. *Toast*: wholemeal, please. Packed portions of *margarine* and *butter* = 10g.	*Egg sandwich*: choose from supermarket low-calorie or reduced-fat sandwich range Sandwich bar – stipulate no spread on bread and without mayonnaise, if possible. *Apple*	*Salmon steak*, grilled: any fish will do, so long as it is grilled, poached, baked without (too much) fat. Choose boiled, or other, potatoes cooked without fat. Select 2 portions of vegetables. If fish is unavailable, choose lean meat. *V Polenta with spicy/ tomato sauce*: some restaurants offer polenta served with Mediterranean vegetables (e.g. ratatouille). If not, try a vegetarian risotto, paella, pilau. **PUDDING** *Fruit salad*: from supermarkets and on restaurant menus (forgo the cream).
Days 2 & 16	*Grapefruit and prunes*: check both the grapefruit and prunes are unsweetened. Request unsweetened juice. Toast, as day 1.	*Cheese and apple sandwich*: as day 1. *Yogurt*: low fat or 'diet' range.	*Chicken risotto*: if risotto is unavailable, choose a plain cooked chicken (or other lean meat) with vegetables and plain potatoes or plain (e.g. not fried) rice. *V Vegetable risotto*. **PUDDING** *Baked apple*: for an office lunch, choose a piece of fruit. In a restaurant, opt for fruit salad.

	BREAKFAST	LUNCH	DINNER
Days 3 & 17	*Porridge*: ask how they make it. Request it be made with skimmed or semi-skimmed milk or water, and (if in Scotland) easy on the salt, and without double cream, brown sugar and whisky!	*Tomato soup and roll*: make your own soup and take it in a flask. Avoid 'cream of' soups, as these will be higher in fat. Substitute clear vegetable soup if necessary. No spread on the bread roll.	*Avocado and pasta salad*: ask for avocado to be served without the vinaigrette and team it up with salad or vegetables cooked without too much fat. Alternatively, choose a low fat pasta dish. PUDDING *Raisin pancake*: available from most supermarkets. In restaurants, choose a crêpe with a low-fat or fruit filling.
Days 4 & 18	*Fruit juice*: as day 1. *Breakfast cereal*: as day 1. *Banana*: don't limit yourself. If more fresh fruit is available, have some.	*Tuna jacket potato*: avoid tuna and mayonnaise mixes, ask for tuna only on the potato. Moisten with milk, not fat. Office lunch? Buy the baked spud and put your own tuna on. Substitute a sandwich, if necessary (see day 1) *V Cheese jacket potato*: watch the amount of cheese. Choose lower-fat (e.g. cottage) cheese.	*Anchovy pasta*: any pasta dish with a mainly vegetable, low-fat sauce (e.g. not a rich lasagne or cream sauce) would be suitable. *V Spinach gnocchi*: if gnocchi is unavailable, or served with a fatty/creamy sauce, choose pasta (as above). PUDDING *Instant fruit fool*: choose the low-fat version(s) in supermarkets. Ask what the ingredients are in a restaurant, and then decide.

93

BREAKFAST	LUNCH	DINNER

Days 5 & 19

Hot Cross bun: or 2 slices of wholemeal toast with 1 portion spread/jam etc.
Fruit compote: as much as you like. Substitute fresh fruit, if necessary.

Cheese and carrot bap: buy a wholemeal cheese sandwich and grate your own carrot (see other sandwich notes above).

Haddock and prawn fishcake: fishcakes can be bought ready-made from supermarkets. Choose the lowest fat version, serve with additional vegetables.
V Vegetable burger: choose carefully, as many vegetarian burgers are high in fat. Opt for a 'diet' or reduced-fat version.

PUDDING
Blackberry and apple summer pudding: the fruit content may differ, but summer pudding is available from supermarkets and on many restaurant menus.

Days 6 & 20

Fruit juice: as day 1.
Carrot and raisin muffin: choose a similar muffin, or wholemeal toast (as above), avoid croissants and brioche (too fatty).

Hummus, toast and vegetables: office lunch? Buy supermarket salad to accompany hummus, if vegetables unavailable. Hummus sandwich from supermarket is an alternative.

Meatballs in tomato sauce: unless they are 'homemade', these are best avoided as the meat is of unknown quality and they are probably high in fat. Choose a fish meal (day 1) or a lean meat meal (day 2).
V Nutballs: nut cutlets or vegetarian burgers (day 5) are more likely to be available. Check fat content first.

PUDDING
Fruit yogurt: easy enough to buy for an 'office' lunch. In a restaurant, choose something else.

BREAKFAST	LUNCH	DINNER
Days 7 & 21	*Fruit juice*: as day 1. *Carrot and raisin muffin*: as day 6.	*Rollmops on rye*: delicatessens will sell single rollmops. Choose wholemeal bread/roll if rye unavailable. *V Carrot nut salad roll*: most supermarkets sell carrot and nut salad. Buy a separate roll.	*Roast chicken*: remove skin and fat. If roast unavailable, avoid Kiev or breaded or fried. See days 1 and 2. *V Mediterranean Pie*: similar filo pastry 'pie' acceptable but avoid other types of pastry. PUDDING *Apple tart*: see above.

FOOD DIARY for Hotel/B & B/Restaurant: Week 1

Strong Likes: ....

....

....

Strong Dislikes ....

....

....

Aggravations ....

....

....

Emotions ....

	BREAKFAST	LUNCH	· DINNER
Days 8 & 22	*Fruit juice*: see day 1. *Porridge*: see day 3.	*Pan bagna*: *V Pan bagna*: see ciabatta, day 9.	*Seafood lasagne*: if buying ready-meal lasagne, choose lower fat versions where possible. In restaurant, choose pasta with a low-fat fish (meat/vegetarian) sauce. *V Pepper and spinach lasagne*: as above. PUDDING *Fruit kebab*: substitute a piece of fruit, or fruit salad (no cream).
Days 9 & 23	*Grapefruit and prunes*: see day 2. TIP: buy snack-size packs of prunes for overnight bag or handbag. *Toast*: see day 1.	*Tuna ciabatta*: order from sandwich bar, or buy similar from supermarket. Wholemeal sandwich is acceptable alternative (see sandwich, day 1). *V Mozzarella ciabatta*: as above.	*Chicken stir-fry*: in a Chinese restaurant, choose a simple stir-fry accompanied by plain, boiled or steamed rice. Supermarkets sell chilled and frozen versions. *V Quorn stir-fry*: as above. PUDDING *Fruit crunch*: for an office lunch, buy a low-fat, fruited fromage frais. In a restaurant, fruit salad.
Days 10 & 24	*Fruit juice* *Muesli* *Toast*: see day 1.	*Waldorf salad*: as an office lunch, buy a ready-made salad from supermarket or salad bar (no dressing, or low no-fat dressing). In a restaurant, order as above.	*Mackerel Kebabs*: choose any grilled/oven-baked fish from the menu (e.g. salmon, trout, tuna) and plain boiled rice or new potatoes. *V Nut shish kebab*: see day 6. PUDDING *Raisin pancake*: as day 3.

BREAKFAST	LUNCH	DINNER
Days 11 & 25 *Fruit juice*: as day 1. *Breakfast cereal*: as day 1. *Banana*: as day 4.	*Turkey sandwich*: see sandwich, day 1. *V Bean tortilla*: for office lunch, buy ingredients from supermarket.	*Calzone/pizza turnovers*: substitute a small- or medium-sized pizza with a low-fat topping, such as simple marinara (seafood without cheese) or romana (tomato and anchovies). Avoid pepperoni and other fatty meats and toppings with too much cheese. Vegetarians opt for napoletana (tomato, cheese, herbs) without the anchovies, or margherita (tomatoes, mozzarella, parmesan). PUDDING *Coeur à la crème*: substitute low-fat fruited yogurt or fromage frais.
Days 12 & 26 *Hot Cross bun*: as day 5. *Fruit compote*: as day 5.	*Black bean and corn soup and roll*: substitute suitable soup (see day 3).	*Fish steak, tortilla and salsa*: unless you are in a Mexican restaurant, opt for plain fish (see day 1). *V Rösti*: it's unlikely you will find this recipe in a restaurant, so choose as wisely as possible! See previous notes. PUDDING *Trifle*: most restaurant trifle is far too high in fat and sugar. Choose fruit salad or, for a treat, summer pudding (no cream).

BREAKFAST	LUNCH	DINNER
Days 13 & 27	*Fruit juice*: as day 1. *Savoury breakfast croissant*: substitute with a wholemeal muffin, or wholemeal toast (as above). Avoid 'real' croissants and other continental breakfast specialities (too fatty and sugary).	*Chicken and coleslaw sandwich*: office lunch? Buy supermarket version or buy ready-cooked chicken piece, remove skin and serve with low calorie coleslaw (see also sandwich, day 1). *V Bruschetta*: substitute French stick (white or wholemeal) for the toast.	*Salad niçoise*: where available on the menu, order without dressing, or dressing 'on the side'. Alternatively, choose a different salad from the menu. *V Scotch egg*: as above. **PUDDING** *Fruit brûlée*: our recipe is nothing like the dieters' double-cream nightmare that constitutes most restaurant and supermarket brûlées, so avoid! It's fruit salad – again . . . or, if you want a treat, choose a frozen yogurt or sorbet.
Days 14 & 28	*Fruit juice*: as day 1. *Savoury breakfast croissant*: as day 13.	*Goat's cheese and rocket salad*: any type of cheese may be used as substitute, but watch the amount. For hard cheese and creamy soft cheeses, piece should be not much bigger than a matchbox! Watercress (or any other salad leaves) will do instead of rocket (no dressing).	*Chicken/rabbit casserole*: you might be lucky, with a lowish fat casserole, or similar dish. However, beware – most restaurant sauces for meat are rich and creamy. Avoid especially fatty casseroles such as cassoulet. *V Minestrone casserole*: opt for a minestrone soup (vegetarian version) and order extra vegetables with it. Some fresh chilled minestrone soups from supermarkets are suitable for vegetarians. **PUDDING** *Orange and mango jelly*: forget the jelly bit, and eat mango and orange as a fruit salad. Vegetarian jelly crystals are acceptable to vegetarians.

FOOD DIARY for Hotel/B & B/Restaurant: Week 2

Strong Likes ....

....

....

Strong Dislikes ....

....

....

Aggravations ....

....

....

Emotions ....

What would you like to drink?

The question that you are most likely to be asked as soon as you enter a restaurant . . . and a comparison of the calories in different drinks.

Aperitifs (pub measures: ⅓ gill (50ml) or small schooner)

Dubonnet Dry	55
Martini Extra Dry	55
Noilly Prat	55
Dry sherry	55
Medium sherry	60
Cream sherry	65
Dubonnet Red	75
Martini Bianco	75
Martini Rosso	80
Cinzano Bianco	80
Pimms No 1	95
Campari	115

Spirits (pub measures: ⅙ gill (25ml))

Whisky	50
Gin, rum, vodka 70°	50
80°	60

Mixers (pub measure: ⅚ gill (125ml))

Low-calorie bitter orange, lemon	5–15
Dry ginger	14
Bitter lemon	35
American ginger ale	39
Lemonade	40
Tonic	40

Wine

Dry white	75
Rosé	80
Dry red	80
Sparkling white	90
Sweet red	95
Sweet white	100

Liqueurs (pub measure: ⅙ gill (25ml))

Calvados	60
Cherry brandy	65
Strega	75
Tia Maria	75
Crème de menthe	80
Grand Marnier	80
Baileys Original Irish Cream	85
Cointreau	85
Drambuie	85
Benedictine	90
Chartreuse (green)	100

Unsweetened fruit juice (pub measures: ⅚ gill (125ml))

Tomato	20
Grapefruit	35
Orange	40
Pineapple	55

Mineral water	0

Takeaway Swaps – *lower calorie choices at your local takeaway.*

CHINESE

Starter or side dish
Usual – Spare ribs in barbecue sauce 300g
Total 550–850cal
Swap – Spring roll 200g, or fried egg roll 115g
Total 400–575cal
Saving 150–275cal

Main meal
Usual – Sweet and sour pork or beef 150–325g
Total 700–1,000cal
Swap – Beef or chicken chow mein 150–325g
Total 400–500cal
Saving 200–600cal

INDIAN

Usual – Lamb rogan josh, biryani or similar red meat curry 200g
Total 900cal
Usual – chicken curry such as chicken madras 200g
Total 800cal
Swap – Chicken tikka masala, or similar dry cooked meat curry 200g
Total 345cal
Saving 455–555cal

CHINESE/INDIAN RICE

Usual – Special fried rice 225g
Total 550–800cal
Usual – Pilau rice 225g
Total 400cal
Swap – Steamed or boiled rice 225g
Total 250cal
Saving 150–550cal

GREEK

Usual – Donner kebab and salad 225g
Total 750cal
Swap – Shish kebab and salad 225g
Total 500cal
Saving 250cal

PIZZA

Usual – Large deep dish pizza 400–450g
Total 800–1400cal
Swap – Medium thin crust pizza 250g
Total 500–650cal
Saving 300–750cal

BURGER

Usual – Halfpounder, or two burgers in bun with cheese
Total 750–900cal
Swap – Plain burger in bun or quarterpounder with relish
Total 260–400cal
Saving 400–500cal

FRIES AND CHIPS

Usual Thin cut French fries 150g
Total 475cal
Swap – Thick cut chips 150g
Total 430cal
Saving 45cal

Takeaway Safety Advice When using cook-chill meals, get them home quickly and put them in the fridge straight away. Keep them refrigerated (check your fridge's temperature, which should be 5°C or below) until ready for use. Check the use by date. Ensure you reheat ready meals (and takeaways, where applicable) until piping hot, especially if using a microwave oven.

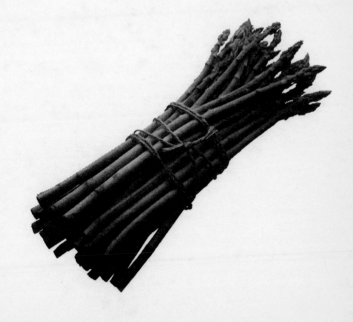

Chapter 5

Problem Solving

There are often difficulties that get in the way before you can start to improve your diet. There are also myths about why you are overweight, and there are personal beliefs and prejudices that may be stopping you setting out on the road that will lead to an easier relationship with food, and yourself.

Many of the myths and misconceptions are outlined below. Some of them will relate to you, your weight problems and experiences of dieting. The solutions to these specific problems are also there for you to read – and to try for yourself, because the answers to your weight problems are in your hands.

We offer no apologies for some of the frank (you might think brutal) facts that follow. They are there so that you do not waste any more time, money and effort in following the wrong diet and the wrong advice.

'To curb those raging appetites that are
Most disobedient and refractory'
    (*Troilus and Cressida*, ii, ii, 181–182)

Being slim is just a fashion. I don't need to lose weight

Women are generally more concerned about being overweight than men. Most women view being even moderately overweight as a 'bad thing'. However, some dismiss slimness as mere fashion. It is not. There are good health reasons not to be overweight. Obesity increases your risk for coronary heart disease, certain cancers, diabetes, gall stones, hypertension (high blood pressure) and range of bone, joint and skin disorders. The more overweight you are, the greater the risk.

It's not my fault that I am overweight. I have a slow metabolic rate

A proportion of overweight people think there is something wrong with their bodies and that they are overweight because of metabolic problems (or hormonal, see below). They believe they are different from other people, as far as their weight is concerned. They think they eat less than people who are not overweight. And they believe it is impossible for them to lose weight by their own efforts.

They are wrong. Studies have shown that overweight people do not have lower metabolic rates than normal weight people. They simply eat more. They may protest that they do not, but they consistently under-record their food intake by astonishing amounts. This means that there is no justification for blaming weight problems on metabolism – except for a few rare diseases (see below).

In fact, overweight people have a higher resting metabolism than normal-weight people because of their greater body size. They may have slightly smaller metabolic rate responses to food (known as dietary thermogenesis) but this does not have a significant impact on the number of calories they burn every day. So they will not put on more weight than a normal weight person eating the same (or correct) amount of food.

I don't eat a thing, and yet I still put on weight

Really?! Many overweight people have a history of bingeing. Not of the type associated with bulimia, but more similar to the way some Celts like to drink – to excess on one or two nights a week. Whatever you tell us about your eating habits, the truth is overweight people consistently under-record their food intake. Is this a genuine mistake or a deliberate attempt to cover up their embarrassment about the amount they eat? You tell us.

I can't lose weight. I'm just made this way. It's my genes!

So, you think you are overweight because your weight problems are genetically determined. You think some people are born fat and therefore there is nothing you can do about it. You are also wrong. Genetic influences may account for 35 per cent of differences in BMI (page 43), mainly in later life.

An obesity gene has been found in mice. Mice given the obesity gene – or rather the obesity protein called leptin – lost weight and maintained a lowered weight by reduced appetite and increased activity and metabolism. But no identical gene has so far been found in humans. However, there is a gene that is 84 per cent identical with the mouse obesity gene and it may interfere with the natural appetite, resulting in a defective satiety response. People affected by it might not feel full up, or satisfied with what they have eaten, in the same way that normal weight people do. So they carry on eating, leading to obesity. But the good news is you can adjust your eating habits to prevent, or treat, obesity. You can also take more exercise (page 39). So there *is* quite a lot you can do about your genetic tendencies.

Genetic mutations in humans may also disrupt the appetite/satiety system and may possibly slightly reduce resting metabolic rate, resistance to insulin and make people susceptible to putting on weight around their tummies. But the good news is, that even if you have one or all of these inherited tendencies, weight problems are not inevitable. The right diet, lifestyle and environment can all be used to counteract these tendencies. Quite a lot of positive things can be done to prevent or treat your weight problems.

I only put on weight since I got married ... had children ...

'... O curse of marriage,
That we can call these delicate creatures ours,
And not their appetites!'
  (*Othello*, III, iii, 268–70)

A large number of people blame their weight problems on an incident in their lives which is really an ordinary occurrence that does not lead to weight problems in other people. A few examples of what these people tell us include: 'I've *suddenly* become fat during or after an illness, or during pregnancy, or on taking the pill, or as a result of the menopause, or as a result of inevitable middle-age spread.' According to these people, quite ordinary life stages are to blame for their eating habits. Marriage meant they no longer had to work so hard at staying in shape to be attractive (not a very nice compliment to their partners!); or that they ate more because they were at home more often – for example, while watching TV in the evenings; or their more structured routine and settled habits meant bigger and more regular meals.

Parenthood is given as an excuse for weight problems by some. Becoming a parent gave them more to worry about than their looks. They tended to nibble when they were at home with the children and during the preparation of regular meals for their children. They also had to eat up the children's leftovers!

The truth is that this group is treating the ordinary as if it were special and using it as an escape from, and an excuse for not, taking responsibility for weight problems they have created themselves. Their metabolic rate will cope well with changes in weight at different stages in their lives such as infancy, pregnancy, adolescence, and even during the menstrual cycle without long-lasting weight problems. Any permanent weight gain must be due to overeating. Once again, there is plenty these people can do to change their weight and shape – once they take the responsibility.

I can't lose weight. The stress of my job means I eat more and I don't have time for exercise and all that

Certain jobs may mean more responsibility, possibly more entertaining and eating out. If a job means working longer hours, then it is even more important to build in breaks and time for exercise. Physical activity helps reduce stress levels and re-energizes you so that you can carry on working for longer. The important thing is to find an activity you like and that is convenient enough to fit into your work and lifestyle. For strategies on eating out without putting on weight, see page 89.

I blame it all on chocolate. I can't live without it

A sizeable group of people with a weight problem blame it on their addiction to chocolate. Hardly surprising, because Britain is the largest confectionery market in Europe, worth £4.5 billion a year, of which we spend £3.1 billion on chocolate. This means your natural appetite is up against £100 million worth of advertising a year, spent by the confectionery market on trying to persuade you into more than 150,000 outlets selling confectionery. Consider how many of the following places selling confectionery also offer you the option of fresh fruit or other 'healthier' snacks: confectioners, newsagents, tobacconists, supermarkets, service stations and convenience stores. It's no wonder that the 'average' Briton eats more than half a pound (268g to be precise) of confectionery per week, which converts to spending £77 per person per year. Of course you do not have to give up chocolate, it can be an occasional treat (see how to balance your diet chart, page 34). Next time you are tempted, think of how else you could spend that money. Do you really want to give more of your money to top brands like KitKat (worth over £210 million a year) owned by Nestlé and subject of a long-standing boycott organized by Baby Milk Action, followed by Mars, Cadbury's Dairy Milk, Roses and Twix (all £145 million)? And, incidentally, chocoholics' addiction is only psychological – it's not a real addiction, so you can give it up, or enjoy it as a treat.

I put on weight when I gave up smoking

That may be so, but it need not be so. You can quit without weight gain. Not everyone puts on weight when they stop smoking. For those who do, it is usually only a few pounds, which can be lost within a matter of months once you are feeling more comfortable with the way you look and eat. The reason some people put on a bit of weight is that smoking depresses the appetite and reduces the sensation of taste. The body also burns calories trying to detoxify itself from the poisonous by-products of smoking. The main thing is to be positive. You will be healthier and look better once you have given up. As this book shows, you can control your weight through exercise and diet – and without smoking. You probably will not have to eat less – just differently. Call Quitline on 0800 002200.

I take the feminist view – it's fine to be fat. I'm happy with the way I look and my partner likes me this way

We take your point. You have good reason to complain that women are pressurized to be unreasonably thin. We don't want you to look like a supermodel stick-insect. But there are health risks associated with being overweight and obese. If your partner happens to have a penchant for plump women, that's fine, but you should equally be aware that it is a feminist myth that it's fine to be fat.

I don't agree with the tables the experts work out for BMIs

'Belike then my appetite was not princely got'
   (2 Henry IV, ii, ii, 11)

They take too little account of important physiological differences between individuals, especially men. Many men fudge the issue of being overweight. To those who do, being 'big' equates with strength and manliness. Moderately overweight men often refuse to acknowledge they have a problem. They think slimming is for women.

OK, if that's the way they want to play it, then they should get fit, rather than going on a diet. They might then find that they get fitter even quicker by modifying the type and amount of food (and drink) they consume. Of course, the real masochists (the ones who enjoy a triple vindaloo with chilli poppadams on the side) will prefer an extreme crash (very low calorie) diet – probably so that they can return to their 'normal' eating (and drinking) habits as quickly as possible.

Someone is going to have to try to get it into their heads that successful slimming is about gradual and long-term changes in diet and lifestyle. Good luck!

I can't do it on my own and slimming clubs are a rip-off

We have spoken to some members of slimming clubs who resent the fact that clubs are commercial businesses. They see them as exploiting fat people. Other people take the view that some clubs are naïve and patronizing. Slimmers think they set unrealistically low target weights to promote longer-term attendance (to boost profits for the clubs). If that is your attitude, then you really are going to have to do it for yourself.

The good news is that you are not alone. Even without a club, you can do it with the help of this book. Get together with a group of friends or like-minded people and encourage each other by meeting regularly for mutual support and assistance. Put up a notice (with permission) in your family doctor's surgery, or in the canteen at work, or at your children's school, or church hall to recruit your own 'members'.

What I really need to help me lose weight is more help . . . pills from the doctor . . . more willpower . . . free access to leisure centres for overweight people . . . my employer to take a health initiative in the canteen . . .

What you *are* asking for is someone else to lose weight for you. It is not a job you can delegate. If you seriously want drugs, we would try to dissuade you. Amphetamine-like appetite suppressants (slimming aid pills) have narrowly escaped a ban by the Department of Health. They may be addictive; some have side-effects that affect speech, mobility and the mind. And they do not help in the long term. What you have to recognize is that your weight problem came about gradually, possibly through years of overeating little and often. Regular chocolate habits, regular snacking between meals, regularly eating up the leftovers when you were actually already feeling rather full . . . and so on. There is no instant weight loss that will last forever on offer from anyone. All you need do is accept that you could just as easily see the weight fall off again in exactly the same way – gradually. Adjusting your eating habits, so that you are no longer regularly overeating little and often, will mean a slow weight loss, but it will be a permanent one. Meanwhile, carry on campaigning for free access to leisure centres for the overweight and lobby your place of work to provide healthier choices in the canteen.

I'll lose weight – later

Virtually everyone who is overweight wants to look slimmer. But many overweight people have no immediate or compelling reason to lose weight (rather like smokers who think they will be able to give up when they really want to). In the meantime, the weight continues to gradually increase, which this group of people do not regard as a problem – certainly not one seen as affecting health. They associate the health risks of being overweight with the obese or elderly. They convince themselves they would get warning of any serious impending trouble, which would then motivate them to lose weight. They are wrong. The heart attack, maturity onset diabetes, arthritis or other health problems will hit them first – and then it may be too late.

I'm waiting for a painless way to lose weight

> 'Appetite, an universal wolf, So doubly seconded with will and power'
>   *Troilus and Cressida*, (I, iii, 121–2)

The painless diet is the one sought by most overweight people who want rapid success without much effort on their part. But how can they expect an overnight solution when the obesity itself has not developed overnight? The plain, but unpalatable, truth is that painless solutions are impossible.

Often the most attractive idea to people seeking the painless way is the easiest, and this is a very low calorie diet in the form of liquid-meal replacements for several weeks. If they have the willpower to stick to it, weight loss will result, but the method does nothing to re-educate the appetite of the person or teach them how to eat well in the long term so, in the long term, it fails.

There are other 'painless' ways to lose weight. You can pay beauty therapists large sums of money to rub cellulite-reducing creams and fat mobilizing gels on to your thighs and stomachs. They will then leave you to sweat it out in a space suit or sauna and afterwards measure your thighs and tell you how much fat you have lost. This is just a trick of the trade. You will actually have lost only a little water in the process. Fat will only be burned off if beauty therapies are done in conjunction with effective aerobic exercise and changes to diet.

You can also pay a hypnotherapist for the pleasure of sitting in his or her comfy chair while he or she whittles away your inches by programming your psyche not to give in to hunger. Alternatively, you can buy hypnosis tapes to play while you sleep. You can also take herbal supplements to help you slim. You might enjoy these 'treatments', but they will only work if, in conjunction, you put in the effort to adjust what you eat and take the right amount of physical activity.

I've tried dieting before, and it doesn't work

You have a pessimism barrier that is hard to remove. Your experience of slimming diets has been a lot of self-denial, followed by putting all the weight back on once the diet is over. You see any further attempts to lose weight as denial extending into an indefinite future. You are put off by slimming diets that in the past have meant thinking about and modifying what you normally eat. You see this as disrupting personal and family eating patterns. Most of these problems have been caused by following the wrong type of slimming diet in the past, which has failed to address the other imbalances that underlie wrong eating habits.

I like dieting. I don't want to give it up – I like trying new diets!

You are the kind of woman (usually) who enjoys a bizarre, gimmicky slimming diet. You believe the half-truths, homespun hypotheses and quackery that surrounds the change to an abnormal diet. You think it's great, mainly because it is only temporary. Once you have lost weight, you can get back to your old habits! The only trouble is, each time you go on a new diet, the weight is more difficult to lose and you seem to put on more between diets. This is part of the vicious circle of Yo-Yo dieting (page 10). After all, if the first diet you tried had worked, you would not have had to try another, and another. Far better to adopt a pattern of eating and lifestyle that will maintain your weight in the long term – and free your time so that you can find an alternative hobby to dieting.

I already eat a healthy diet, so I don't need to make any changes. I don't lose weight because I'm just made this way

People tend to overestimate their consumption of healthy foods and underestimate their consumption of unhealthy foods. They especially underestimate their fat intake. Despite thinking we eat a healthier diet today, fat consumption remains constant, at about 40 per cent of energy derived from food. Thus, we underestimate the risks we face from nutrition and weight-related problems; a pattern of findings replicated in many pieces of research.

HOW TO UNDERSTAND AND TACKLE PROBLEMS THAT ARISE WHEN DOING THE DIET

In addition to changes in your food desires, aversions and aggravations, and emotional changes that may arise from altering your diet, there are a number of other potential problems that require understanding.

What does it mean if I develop headaches or feel unwell during the first few days of the diet?

If your diet has been very different to the Natural Appetite diet and you start it abruptly, the body's metabolism will have to quickly readjust to the loss of some items of food that it is used to and the intake of others that it is unused to dealing with. Normally, this process takes place very quickly and without much problem. Headaches in the first few days are very often a result of caffeine withdrawal, particularly if you have been drinking a lot of tea, coffee or cola-based drinks before starting the diet. These usually settle very quickly, but if they are bad, you may need to take a homeopathic remedy or a painkiller. If they persist and you have been on a high caffeine intake, go back to your original levels of caffeine and reduce more slowly.

General feelings of fatigue and being unwell in the first few days of the diet are usually just a readjustment and should pass quickly. They may be associated with the withdrawal of foods that you have an intolerance to and, therefore, addiction to. This is a withdrawal effect and should quickly pass. If it does persist, go back on your original diet. Try to identify, by means of elimination and challenge, which food is responsible, then cut it down more slowly.

What does it mean if I start to suffer from a sudden loss of energy or cold, shaky, hyped-up feelings?

These symptoms are very suggestive of a drop in your blood sugar (hypoglycaemia). They probably mean that you were eating fairly high quantities of unrefined carbohydrates before starting the diet and, although these have been removed, your pancreas is still producing high amounts of insulin and has not yet readjusted to the lower levels of refined carbohydrates in the Natural Diet. The simplest course of action is to have small, frequent, non-sugar-based snacks, say every two hours, so that you have eaten before the drop in blood sugar occurs. You can then increase the duration of time between the snacks until you are eating to your preferred schedule.

I feel better for doing the diet but have noticed that I have developed some new symptoms or some of my old symptoms have got worse.

When you are on the Natural Diet, every cell in your body will start to function more efficiently. Very often the body takes advantage of this to do a 'spring-clean' and to try to put into balance those functions of the body which have been malfunctioning. This may lead to a temporary worsening of symptoms that have been there previously, or you may develop a runny nose or new symptoms, which is the body's way of eliminating toxins. Providing you are feeling better in yourself and these do not last for more than a few days, just accept them. If they persist or if you are also feeling unwell, you may have a medical problem.

What happens if I go on the diet and I have a genuine medical problem?

Although a genuine medical condition rarely accounts for weight gain, as we have said before, should you feel that your general health is compromised, it would be sensible and prudent to have a medical examination and advice from your family doctor before attempting the Natural Diet. Some of the medical conditions which do include weight gain as part of the picture include:

Hypothyroidism – This is a condition where the thyroid gland is not producing enough thyroxine to keep the metabolic rate at its desired level. Symptoms, apart from the weight gain, include always feeling cold, constipation, thinning hair and dry skin.

Cushing's Syndrome – This is most common in young and middle-aged women and is due to an overproduction of steroids by the adrenal glands, possibly as a result of an adrenal or pituitary tumour, or as a side-effect of long-term steroid treatment. Features include a moon-faced look, muscle wasting and easy bruising.

Fluid retention – This can also be due to kidney or heart disease. It is also common in women who suffer from premenstrual syndrome.

Drugs – Some drugs are notorious for putting on weight, especially steroids and oral contraceptives.

What does it mean if I develop indigestion or bowel problems?

Whilst the Natural Diet is one that most doctors and health educators would love to see everybody in the nation on, some people do have problems with handling the new types of food in the diet. Indigestion (hiccoughs, belching, discomfort after eating, heartburn, chest pain, stomach ache, acidity or wind) can be caused by, amongst other things, citrus fruits, fruit skins, cooked cabbage, tomatoes, onions, cucumbers, beans, pulses, nuts, bread, pork, spices and foods not found in the Natural Diet, e.g. wine, neat spirits, fizzy drinks. Eating too much at once or too quickly, or swallowing air while eating, can also result in indigestion. It may be due to anxiety, too, connected with the diet, as may irritable bowel syndrome, the main symptoms of which are alternating constipation and diarrhoea, sometimes with cramping lower abdominal pains and pain on passing stools. The most common foods likely to cause irritable bowel syndrome are wheat, corn, dairy products, citrus fruit, tea, coffee, apples, pears and salads.

In all these examples, a process of elimination and challenge should be used to identify which foods are responsible and, of course, these should be noted down in the 'aggravation' section of the diary.

How can I avoid becoming anorexic or bulimic if I change my diet?

The Natural Diet is *not* a crash diet to make you lose lots of weight quickly, it is to enable you to achieve a pattern of eating for life. Both anorexia and bulimia are to do with the state of your mind and emotions rather than the actual food that you eat. It is highly unlikely that doing the Natural Diet for one month will precipitate either of these conditions unless the potential for them already exists. You have no need to worry unless you find that, during the course of doing the diet, you become obsessional about calories and try to maintain your weight too low, or become fixated on your appearance and think that you are more overweight than you really are. These are the main symptoms of anorexia – should they develop, even to a slight degree, you should abandon the diet and seek medical help.

Similarly, if you develop a desire to vomit after food and then binge, or use laxatives to try to get rid of the food you have eaten, you should again abandon the diet immediately and seek medical help, as these are the main features of developing bulimia.

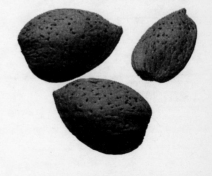

Chapter 6

Finding Your Homeopathic Food Type

By now hopefully you will have completed your 28-day Natural Diet and completed the Food Diary in which you will have noted down your likes, dislikes and aggravations to food, and a note of your emotional state. (And any other major changes you have noticed in yourself, such as experiencing an increase in body temperature, etc.) If you have not managed to complete the entire 28-day diet, don't worry, as long as you have written down your initial emotional state and food information.

If you have completed it, it will be obvious to you that any likes, dislikes, aggravations or strong emotions that have remained unchanged at the end of the 28-day diet are the most significant ones. But if, at the end of the diet, you still feel you are not in balance and in touch with your natural appetite, then we can use the information that you put down at the beginning of the diet, and any changes that have occurred during the diet, and use those.

Now you need to know how to use all this information in order to find a homeopathic remedy that will restore you to balance and put you back in contact with your natural appetite, thus helping you, along with a sensible eating plan and exercise, to achieve your natural weight. Before we do this, however, there are three golden rules that have to be understood. Please make sure you have read Chapter 2 before proceeding.

I The homeopathic remedy you need may not be in this book

This book mentions only the twelve remedies that Dr Lockie and a colleague have found most commonly used in weight problems in a survey of patients in his practice. There are scores, if not hundreds, more remedies that can be used, so don't worry if you do not fit neatly into one of the food types.

2 Only use a remedy if the picture is very clear

We will discuss this again later, but it may be that you are unable to decide between two or more remedies for a variety of reasons. Firstly, as mentioned above, the remedy you need may not be present; secondly, you may have insufficient information to go on; thirdly, it is quite difficult to observe oneself carefully enough sometimes to find the right remedy; and fourthly, you may have a more complex imbalance than can be treated by self-help methods. Remember, the more imbalances that exist in your will, intellect or emotions, or the more severe your physical symptoms, the less able you will be to help yourself. In all of these cases, it is best to see a skilled homeopath.

3 Always follow the rules for prescribing remedies

This is dealt with in detail later.

How to use the charts

Food Information

On a piece of paper write down all your strong likes, strong dislikes and aggravations. Now turn to the charts and you will find that there are three corresponding sections, under which are a list of foods and next to which are a series of numbers with the name of a homeopathic remedy above them.

The number represents the strength of that symptom for that particular remedy – for example, if you look at Strong likes, Alcohol, which is the first item, Sulph., Ars. and Lach. are all a 3. This represents a very strong liking for alcohol. Puls., Phos., Lyc., Calc. and Sep. are all a 2, which represents a moderate liking, and Nat-m. and Merc. are both a 1, which represents only a slight liking, whereas Caust. and Kali-c. have no score, which means that people requiring these remedies do not often have a liking for alcohol at all. It may mean that they have a strong dislike, but if you look at Strong dislikes, Alcohol, you will find that Caust. and Kali-c. again have no score, so people requiring these two remedies have neither a strong liking, nor a strong dislike, for alcohol. On the other hand, Ars. and Merc. have slightly and moderately strong dislikes for alcohol respectively.

This may seem strange at first, but it is entirely possible for the person requiring a particular homeopathic remedy either to have a strong dislike for a food or drink, or a strong liking for it. Equally, when you look at the first entry in Aggravations, Alcohol, all the remedies except for Kali-c. have some degree of aggravation from alcohol. Again, this is not a contradiction as it is entirely possible to have a strong liking for alcohol, but also to be aggravated or upset by it.

Turn to your list of strong likes, strong dislikes and aggravations, and work through the columns, circling every remedy that appears under the food or drink that you have written down. At the end, you total them all up; the remedies with the highest scores are the ones that are most likely to represent your type. For example, if you have written down that you have a strong liking for hard-boiled eggs and sweets, but you don't like milk and in fact it upsets you, as does dry food and flatulence-causing food, then circle all the remedies that are mentioned under those headings and total up the score.

You will find that Calc. comes out top at 16, Lyc. at 13 and Puls., Sulph. and Sep. have 10 each. It is therefore most likely that the remedy that might suit you will be one of these five. Make a note of these remedies and then look at the information that you have written down under the emotions heading.

STRONG LIKES	Puls.	Sulph.	Phos.	Lyc.	Calc.	Sep.	Ars.	Nat. m.	Lach.	Merc.	Caust.	Kali. c.
Alcohol	2	3	2	2	2	2	3	1	3	1		
Bitter-tasting food						1	2	2				
Bitter drinks						1	2	2				
Bread	2			1			2	2		2		
Cold water, icy			2					2				
Cold food (any food at all, as long as it is cold)	3		3	2			2	1	1	2	1	
Cucumber	2		2									
Eggs and egg dishes	2				2							
Fruit juices	1		1				2				1	
Ice cream	1	1	3		2			1				
Lemonade	1				1				1			
Lemons	1						1	1		2		
Meat					2	1	1	1		1	1	
Meat, smoked											3	

STRONG LIKES

	Puls.	Sulph.	Phos.	Lyc.	Calc.	Sep.	Ars.	Nat. m.	Lach.	Merc.	Caust.	Kali. c.
Milk	1	2	2		2		2	2	1	2		
Milk, cold		2	2									
Raw food or salads		3			1							
Salt		1	3		2			3		1	2	
Sauerkraut								2			3	
Sausages	1										3	
Smoked Food	1							1			3	
Soup		2						1		1		
Soured foods, e.g. vinegar, sour cream	2	3	2		2	2	2	2	2			2
Warm drinks		2		2			3					1
Warm food (any food as long as it is warm)				2			3					

STRONG DISLIKES	Puls.	Sulph.	Phos.	Lyc.	Calc.	Sep.	Ars.	Nat. m.	Lach.	Merc.	Caust.	Kali. c.
Alcohol		1	1	1	1		1			2		
Beans and peas		3		2				1				
Bread	3	1	2	2	2	2		1	2			3
Fish		1	2					1				
Fruit	3		1				3	1			2	
Garlic			2									
Hot drinks	2			1							1	
Pastry dishes	2		2	1			2					
Pork	2					1						
Potatoes			2			1						
Puddings			2		1		1					
Salt	1		1	1		2		2		2		
Sausages	1						2					
Soured foods, e.g. vinegar, sour cream		2		1				1				
Starchy food		2		1								

AGGRAVATIONS	Puls.	Sulph.	Phos.	Lyc.	Calc.	Sep.	Ars.	Nat. m.	Lach.	Merc.	Caust.	Kali. c.
Alcohol	2	2	2	2	2	1	3	2	3	2	2	
Beans and peas	1	1	1	3	2	1	1	1				1
Bread	3	2	1	2		2		2		1	2	1
Bread and butter	3	1	1			2		1				
Buckwheat	3		2			2						
Eggs	3	2		1	2							
Fatty foods	3	2	1	2	1	2	2	1		1	2	1
Fish	2			1		1	1		1			1
Fish, shell-				2								
Flatulence-causing food	1			3	1	1	1	1				
Oysters	2			3								
Pancakes	3										2	

AGGRAVATIONS	Puls.	Sulph.	Phos.	Lyc.	Calc.	Sep.	Ars.	Nat. m.	Lach.	Merc.	Caust.	Kali. c.
Pastry dishes	3	1	2	2			1					2
Pork	3					3	1	2			1	
Potatoes	2	2			1	2						
Raw food or salads	2	1		1	2	1	1		1			
Rich food, e.g.	2	1		1	1	1	1		1			
Christmas pudding												
Starchy foods	3	1		1			1	3	2		2	2
Vegetables				1	1		1					2
Vinegar	2	2	1			2	2	1	1		1	
Warm drinks	2	2	2			1			2			
Warm food	3	1	3		1	1	1	1	3	1	1	2
Wine		2	1	3	2		3	2	2	2		

Your emotions

If, as a result of having done your 28 day diet, you feel well, full of energy, emotionally balanced and at peace with the world, then it is most likely that any physical, emotional and general information that you noted in the diary were simply due to bad diet and if you now go on to the maintenance programme, you should gradually find yourself achieving your ideal weight and maintaining your vitality. If you have not, then it is time to look in more detail at the remedy pictures to see if any of the five remedies that have come out top from your food list, match you in more general terms. For instance, if you have noted down that you have a tendency to eat when worried, that you suffer from panic attacks and depression, that you have a feeling of weakness if you don't eat regularly, and that in addition you have noticed that since doing your diet, you have become more chilly with a tendency to perspire on the back of your neck and head whilst asleep, and if in addition you are prone to have an itchy scalp, stress incontinence which is worse on coughing, and swollen breasts before periods, then it is highly likely that Calc. will be the remedy for you. You should now turn to page 130 for further information.

Please note that you do not have to have all the symptoms that are mentioned in the remedy pictures, but the strongest food information and emotions should be present. The closer they are, the more likely the prescription is to work. If none of them fit, or you cannot choose between two or three of the remedies, you will need help from a homeopath (see page 137).

Remedy Pictures

The following pictures of remedies are simply thumbnail sketches based on information supplied by patients. So, for example, the Pulsatilla Remedy picture contains a description of 'putting on weight even if you only eat small quantities'. *This is how the patient perceives the situation.* The pictures will give you some more information to help you choose the right remedy. They are by no means comprehensive and for further information you should consult a guide to homeopathy (see page 172). If you are still unsure, you will probably need to see a homeopathic practitioner.

Symptom guide

By physical symptoms, we mean symptoms that may be present along with the difficulty in losing weight; by general symptoms, we mean symptoms that apply to you generally in terms of your physical reactions to the environment.

Calcarea

Calcarea (Calc.) types tend to eat when worried, and to be very shy about your weight and very sensitive. Going on a diet like the Natural Diet could bring out feelings of anxiety and worry and you may have a tendency to become obsessive about food to the point where it starts to annoy other people. This in turn will make you feel even more embarrassed and you may be worried that you are going to fail. You may become mildly depressed and very sensitive to scenes of poverty and cruelty in the world around you. You will benefit from lots of reassurance to keep on going, but it will be worth it in the long run.

Physical symptoms: You might have a tendency to feel weak if you do not eat regularly, a tendency to become dizzy, have an itchy scalp, cramping pains, stress incontinence which is worse on coughing, chest pains, stiff neck, clumsiness, eczema, thrush, and both vaginal discharge and swollen breasts before periods.

General symptoms: A tendency to have arthritis and hot flushes. You feel worse in cold weather, and your head has a tendency to profusely sweat into the pillow at night.

Lycopodium

Lycopodium (Lyc.) types tend to put weight on when they are under stress because they eat more when they are anxious and put on weight even when it seems they are eating only small quantities.

Generally, you will appear to be a strong character, but underneath you may well lack confidence and feel very apprehensive about changing your diet. You find it particularly difficult to avoid sweet foods; you may find that going on a diet makes your sexual desire stronger. Whilst it is unlikely that colleagues at work will notice much change in you during the diet, you may tend to become irritable and bad-tempered at home.

Physical symptoms: Difficulty in concentration, dizziness, itchy scalp, falling out of hair, painful eyes, cramping abdominal pains, stress incontinence worse on coughing, breathlessness, stiff neck, sciatica, swelling of the fingers, hot feet, a bloated abdomen and irritability before periods and weepiness before and after periods.

General symptoms: You might have a tendency to arthritis, to feel worse in hot weather and between the times of 4 a.m. and 8 a.m., and 4 p.m. and 8 p.m., to dislike stuffy rooms, and to feel fatigue before periods.

Sepia

Sepia (Sep.) types have a tendency to put on weight under stress, and women during the menopause; it is also very often used where premenstrual tension is a problem. Going on a diet tends to make you irritable and resentful; you hate to be contradicted and will dislike sympathy and tend to become withdrawn. The one thing that will make you feel great in yourself is hard physical exercise like working out or dancing.

Physical symptoms: Difficulty in concentration, hair falling out, stress incontinence worse when laughing or coughing, stiff joints, hot sweats, thrush and vaginal discharge, irritability and fatigue before periods.

General symptoms: A tendency to arthritis, feeling better for warmth, a dislike of cold weather, is stimulated by thunderstorms, may suffer with hot flushes.

Sulphur

Sulphur (Sulph.) types have a tendency to gain weight under stress due to marked increase in appetite, and women especially during the menopause. You tend to think far too much for your own good and can be very intellectual and egotistical. You may become quite stroppy and irritable on the diet, even if you know that it is good for you, and you have a tendency to be lazy and lack willpower and initiative, and not follow the diet through.

Physical symptoms: Itchy scalp, hair falling out, chronic sinusitis, itching in the back passage, stiff joints, swollen fingers, hot feet, hot sweats, eczema, tendency to arthritis, hot flushes and fatigue particularly before periods.

General symptoms: You feel worse in a hot bed and when washing, tend to have an energy drop around 11 a.m., but don't usually feel the cold.

Pulsatilla

Pulsatilla (Puls.) is a remedy for very emotional people; you will tend to readily empathize with others and weep easily and rely on others for support, guidance and advice. You find it difficult to be assertive about changing your diet and to express anger and will tend to avoid confrontation about changing your eating plans just in order to keep the peace. Because of a marked increase in appetite, you put on weight even if you seem only to eat small quantities; it may become worse during the menopause. However, with support from loved ones, you should be able to carry it through.

Physical symptoms: Dizziness, migraines, cramping abdominal pain, stress incontinence worse on laughing or coughing, breathlessness, painful chest, swollen fingers, hot feet, thrush and a bloated abdomen before periods.

General symptoms: Dislike of stuffy rooms, feeling better in the fresh air, marked fluid retention, hot flushes, fatigue particularly before periods, and a tendency to arthritis.

Phosphorus

Phosphorus (Phos.) people tend to be very enthusiastic and will start off the diet full of good intentions; in fact, you will love being the centre of attention as you start to undergo your transformation. Fairly soon, however, you will tend to run out of steam and to become anxious and afraid of failing. Because of a marked increase in appetite, even small quantities of food seem to put on weight. This could lead to you cutting off from people and becoming a bit irritable. However, sympathy and understanding from your loved ones will give you the boost you need and you would respond extremely well to the occasional massage.

Physical symptoms: Dizziness, and fatigue that is worse after periods.

General symptoms: Difficulty in concentration, panic attacks, weepiness before and after periods, dizziness, fatigue which is worse after periods, better for being in the fresh air and for naps, worse before and during thunderstorms.

Lachesis

Going on the Natural Diet will be accompanied by an almost religious zeal, as Lachesis (Lach.) people have a tendency to tell everyone about it, to become suspicious that people are trying to undermine their efforts and to be jealous of others who have succeeded. They also suspect their partners are looking elsewhere to satisfy their affections and may become indecisive and depressed as a result. There may be a weight gain, particularly in the menopause.

Physical symptoms: Hair falling out, sensation of a lump in the throat, breathlessness, stiff neck, painful legs, hot feet, clumsiness and a bloated abdomen, particularly before periods.

General symptoms: Better with the onset of menses or any other discharges, worse for heat, hot flushes, fatigue worse if you have not eaten for a while and also before and after periods.

Natrum muriaticum

Natrum muriaticum (Nat. m.) types have a tendency to put on weight under stress, particularly where there has been a loss or bereavement. Because of a marked increase in appetite, you put on weight even if you seem to eat only a little amount of food. You have a tendency to take the diet very seriously and conscientiously, but may become so self-absorbed in it that you will become moody, despondent, impatient and abrupt. No matter how hard you are finding the diet, your natural extreme sensitivity will make you keep your feelings to yourself; sympathy and help from others will be met by resentment and anger, although inwardly you crave for that understanding. You may become very sensitive to music, which could make you cry.

Physical symptoms: Dizziness, itchy scalp, hair falling out, sore eyes, sensation of a lump in the throat, stress incontinence worse for laughing or coughing, thrush.

General symptoms: Tendency to arthritis, feel worse in hot sunny weather and better for the fresh air, and fatigue and weakness premenstrually.

Kali carbonicum

A patient needing Kali. c. also has a tendency to increasing weight during stress because you eat when you are anxious. A strong sense of duty and high moral standards, associated with a fear of losing control, mean that once you are committed to the diet you will follow it religiously. You may, however, be more sensitive to emotional upset, which characteristically you would feel as a blow to the stomach.

Physical symptoms: Hair falling out, migraines, chronic sinusitis, stiff neck and swollen breasts premenstrually.

General symptoms: You tend to be worse if you have not eaten for a while. Tendency to arthritis. Worse in cold weather, better in warmth. Also worse premenstrually, generally.

Arsenicum album

Arsenicum (Ars.) types eat when they are worried because of their general sense of insecurity in life. You are constantly worried and spend a lot of time planning how to cover eventualities that may occur to protect you against misfortune. With a strong perfectionist streak in you, your approach to the diet may well be all or nothing, and if you cannot follow it absolutely, you may tend to abandon it. During the course of the diet, you may become tense and restless and over-anxious about your own and other people's health and will need constant reassurance from your partners and family, but with their help you can win through.

Physical symptoms: Breathlessness, chest pains, stiff joints, swollen fingers, eczema, marked fluid retention and thrush.

General symptoms: A tendency to exhaustion and to feel the cold. Much better in warm atmospheres.

Causticum

Causticum (Caust.) types eat when worried. Going on the diet may increase your oversensitivity to the suffering of other people. You might also experience the return of sensitivity to previous griefs and sufferings that you have had before in your life. Going on the diet may also make you feel slightly depressed and anxious, overcritical, irritable, suspicious and find it difficult to rely on your own judgement. Just note down these feelings but persevere and you will manage in the long run.

Physical symptoms: Migraines, stress incontinence worse for laughing and coughing, breathlessness, painful chest, stiff neck, stiff joints, hot feeling, clumsiness and irritability before periods.

General symptoms: Tendency to arthritis, worse for dry, cold winds, better for warmth and hot flushes.

Mercurius

Mercurius (Merc.) types tend to overeat when stressed and put on weight when seeming to eat only small quantities. You will probably find that you are very suspicious and cautious about embarking on such a major project as this, because order and stability play a large part in your life. Once you do succeed in going on the diet, you may tend to become restless and anxious and very sensitive to criticism and contradiction, which could lead to you losing your temper if someone offends you. You may also find temporary dulling of your intellect with poor concentration, memory and willpower, but once you have got through this stage, you will feel much better.

Physical symptoms: Painful eyes, swollen fingers and thrush.

General symptoms: Fatigue, tendency to arthritis, worse for extremes of heat and cold with a tendency to perspire and salivate on the pillow at night, and marked fluid retention.

How can I use homeopathy to regain my natural appetite?

By now you should have a very clear idea in your mind of the remedy which most suits your food type and covers your emotions. If the picture is unclear, you probably need further help – see the next section. If you are clear as to what the right remedy is, then you should obtain it in the 30c (which means that the original substance from which the remedy has been made has been diluted and succussed 1:100 and repeated thirty times) potency and take it once a week for up to eight doses.

How to obtain remedies and store them

Homeopathic remedies in the 30c potency may be available in your local chemist or health food shop, or you may have to obtain them from a specialist homeopathic pharmacy (see Useful Addresses, page 176). Remember that homeopathic remedies are not like drugs and are, in fact, subtle messages to the body. This means that they should be stored in a cool, dark place well away from products that have a strong smell, such as mothballs. Please make sure that the tops of the containers are screwed on tightly and remember to keep them well away out of the reach of children, although they are extremely safe; even if a toddler swallowed a whole bottleful, it is most likely he or she would suffer only a slight degree of loose stools as a result of the lactose in the tablets. When stored properly, remedies will last for years.

The next point to observe is that remedies should never be touched by hand. Simply tip a small quantity, about the size of a small fingernail, into the bottom of the lid and put directly on to a clean mouth and tongue. This is because remedies are absorbed directly through the lining of the mouth and do not go into the stomach – in fact, if they do, they are destroyed. The reason for the mouth being clean is twofold: firstly, any food that is present may block the absorption of the remedy and, secondly, strong-tasting food or drink may antidote them. While taking homeopathic treatment, it is advisable to avoid drinking coffee and not to brush the teeth with peppermint toothpaste, at least on the day of taking the remedy.

Reactions to the remedy

Homeopathic remedies act by giving a message to the body to help it to cure itself. Once this message has been delivered, there is no point in carrying on with the remedy – in fact, it can be counter-productive. Thus, although it is said to take it for up to eight weeks, you should stop as soon as you get a reaction, whether good or bad. If you have taken the correct homeopathic remedy, the first thing that you may notice is an increase in vitality and well-being. Your physical symptoms, if you have any, may not improve, but you will feel better in yourself. This will be accompanied by a strengthening of your will, so that you will feel more comfortable about eating according to your natural appetite and you will feel more in tune with yourself. At this point, you should stop taking the remedy, but if you start to feel worse again, you may take another dose. Sometimes it happens that you may feel worse in yourself or, more likely, that any physical symptoms you have may be aggravated. This may well be a sign that the remedy is working and, again, you should stop taking it. Any aggravation from your symptoms will settle down within two to three days. Failure to do so may make you suspect that something else is wrong and you should get a further opinion.

Failure to get any improvement in well-being or symptoms by the end of the last of the eight doses, or an aggravation that is not followed by an improvement, should lead you to seek help from a qualified homeopath.

How to get further help

Unfortunately, at the moment in many countries in the world, the name homeopath applies to at least two different types of practitioner. The first type are medically qualified doctors who have gone on to study homeopathy after completing their basic medical training. In the UK, these doctors are granted the initials MFHom or FFHom by the Faculty of Homeopathy. Homeopaths who are not medically qualified are not usually statutorily regulated, although this varies from country to country; in most countries, it is under review at present. Standards of training in both clinical knowledge and homeopathy vary considerably within the non-medical homeopathic community. In the UK, the Society of Homeopaths give the qualifications RSHom to those homeopaths who they feel have completed enough hours of study and clinical experience to be safe to practise homeopathy.

We would advise that, if you are unable to find a medically qualified homeopath in your area, and you wish to see someone who is not medically qualified, you should remain under the continued care and observation of your own GP.

How to pay for homeopathic treatment

Homeopathic treatment from a doctor working within the National Health Service will, of course, be free. The vast majority of non-doctor homeopaths and a substantial number of doctor homeopaths, however, are in purely private practice. This means that you will have to either pay for the treatment yourself or have it funded by a private health insurance company which recognizes medically qualified homeopathic doctors who have had certain levels of experience and training. Contact your insurance company for more details. It is also now possible for your GP to refer you for homeopathy on the National Health Service in addition to referrals to the five hospitals or NHS clinics.

If your GP is a fund holder, they can pay for this themselves. If they are not, then their local health authority may have a contract with a homeopathic hospital or local practitioners, or your GP could apply to the Local Family Health Services Authority or District Health Authority for special funding. If your GP isn't happy about referring you under the Patients' Charter, you are entitled to ask for a second opinion from a medically qualified homeopathic doctor.

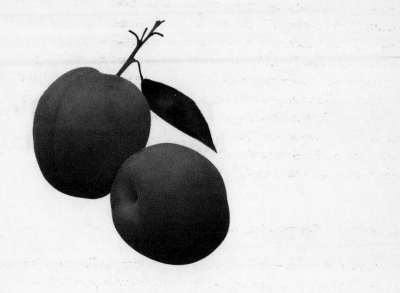

Chapter 7

The Natural Diet
Maintenance Plan

What happens if my cravings return on the maintenance plan?

As we hope you will have understood by now, cravings for particular foods may just be a simple question of the more you eat something, the more you want to eat it and the more your body comes to rely on it, or it may be a symptom of a deeper or more subtle imbalance in your health generally. If you still feel strong in yourself, have plenty of energy and are generally content in your life, it is probable that the craving merely represents slipping into 'bad habits'. If you generally feel out of balance, lack energy, feel your willpower is being eroded and are more emotionally sensitive and vulnerable, or have developed other physical symptoms, then it may be that you need to take your remedy again, or go back and see your homeopathic practitioner.

The easiest way to judge this is to simply deny yourself the foods that you are craving for three or four days. If it is simply a slip into bad habits, you will notice at the end of four days that you have lost the craving. If, however, the craving persists and particularly if you don't feel generally well balanced, this means that something more serious is going on and you need to either take the remedy again or seek further help.

Stay motivated

'But doth not the appetite alter? A man loves the meat in his youth that he cannot endure in his age.'
   (*Much Ado about Nothing*, II, iii, 247)

Staying slim seems like an impossible dream to the habitual dieter. The pounds may fall away at the start of a new diet and they may achieve their perfect body shape and weight – only to wake up weeks or months later, back where they started: an unhappy and dumpy diet failure.

While the Natural Diet cannot promise that you will live happily ever after, it will by now have become clear that it can help you sort out underlying problems with food and allow you to eat a varied balanced diet so that you can comfortably avoid regaining large amounts of weight in future.

Your goal while following the Natural Diet is not to achieve the body of a supermodel, neither is it to transform yourself, through dedication to an impossible diet, into a new person. It is to gently improve your shape and size and gain any associated health benefits. Hopefully, it will also have taught you neither to be ashamed of, nor to dislike, your body (as nine out of ten women are reported to do).

The belief still lingers, however, that, if you change your shape, you will be happier and improve your relationships, because being slim is still an outward sign of being successful and happy, even though it is not natural for women to have flat stomachs, non-existent bottoms and lean thighs. To maintain that shape means starvation; to crash diet produces tiredness, anxiety and unhappiness. Being thin is not the answer, but health, rather than weight, is.

Maintenance will be easier because the diet has not been a crash diet. You do not face the problems that crash dieters do, such as the body depositing energy and fat, especially fat, around the tummy, in case you go on another drastic diet, since it is easier for the body to deposit fat than build muscle.

Following the Natural Diet has helped you change the way you eat, and has explained what makes a healthy diet. From now on you can continue to eat the foods you have enjoyed on the Natural Diet because, unlike crash or restrictive diets, a full range of food and nutrients is incorporated. All you need do is adjust the amount you eat to maintain your weight.

Where do you go from here?

To make the job of weight control easier, it is also vital to ensure you are taking enough exercise. Scientific studies have shown that people who adopt regular physical activity are more likely to sustain a higher percentage of the weight lost through dieting. This is due to a mixture of reasons. Continuing to exercise burns more calories and lean muscle tissue burns more calories than fat. In addition, psychosocial mechanisms seem to be involved.

Activity is very important in preventing a steady slide into becoming overweight with age. Small daily increases in activity levels have significant impact on energy balance over the long term, which means you will never need the emergency measure of a quick-fix crash diet again.

Physical activity is especially useful for men because they tend to store abdominal fat and exercise is the most effective way of removing fat from that area. Building strong tummy muscles will help prevent further weight gain because muscle tissue is metabolically more active. In addition the body is more toned, fitter and feels better.

So what's stopping you?

If the idea of regular exercise is about to make you shut this book and think you have done enough by modifying your diet, please bear with us a little longer. You are not alone in your lack of enthusiasm for physical activity.

Studies show that most men and women stop taking exercise after they leave school. This is often due to dislike of sport or team games, but you need not do these to stay or get fit. Even simple exercise such as walking reduces the risk of things like osteoporosis, which affects one woman in three, later in life.

The four-week maintenance activity plan

Four weeks to get you on the road to fitness.

Week I

The result of relying too much on the car and labour-saving devices, and having sedentary jobs and lifestyles, is not only flabby bodies, but increased risk of heart disease, high blood pressure and other diseases. The aim of your Maintenance Plan is to make exercise a regular part of your life.

You can do it one of two ways. Either, i), choose a strenuous aerobics activity and do three sessions a week, each of which contains a minimum of 20 minutes' work at your full aerobic potential. (For description of aerobic activities, see 'Are you Active or Sedentary?', page 39). Or, ii), go for half an hour's less strenuous physical activity five times a week.

Start now by choosing an activity you enjoy (or think you will enjoy) – for example, swimming or cycling. However, if as a woman you choose either of these, then vary it with another activity such as walking or an aerobics class, which are both weight-bearing exercises, that give protection against osteoporosis.

If you already exercise regularly, start now to perfect your technique. Make sure you are doing movements fully and properly. Do not be misled into trying to keep up with the number and speed of exercises being done by the person next to you in the gym or the aerobics class. Half a dozen properly executed exercises will do you far more good than twice as many incorrect or partially done exercises.

WARNING If exercise is new to you, don't overdo it. 'Going for the burn' is dangerous. Exercise does not have to hurt to do you good. Doing any activity that raises your heart beat and leaves you slightly out of breath is all you need do.

Warm up and cool down correctly

Start your exercise session with some stretching, gentle movement and deep breaths in and out. This avoids injury. You can either do the stretches first, and then walk briskly or use a cycle machine or treadmill for 5 minutes to warm up. Or incorporate the stretches while marching/stepping on the spot for 5–11 mins. After you have finished your 'workout', do not stop immediately. Keep your legs moving gently, e.g. a slow march or gently stepping on the spot, while repeating the stretches.

Week 2

Exercise

You should do either three sessions of your chosen aerobic activity(ies) or five 30-minute (minimum) sessions of moderate or light activity (see page 39).

Aerobics

Vary your chosen activities this week to prevent putting too much strain on the same muscles. For example, make one session jogging, one swimming and one an aerobics class or gym session. This is called cross-training, which professional athletes use to allow different muscles to work and rest on alternate days.

You can do your aerobics at home, either to a video, or try our home workout. 1 Warm up stretches and knee-high marching for 5 minutes. 2 Dancing or running on the spot for 5 minutes. 3 Skipping for 6½ minutes (45 seconds skipping, 45 low stepping while you recover!). 4 Stool stepping or stair climbing for 5 minutes. 5 Repeat steps 2 to 4. 6 Do cool-down stretches while keeping those legs moving.

NB If at any time you feel pain, discomfort or are too breathless, do not stop (unless you are experiencing chest pain), walk around the room gently until you feel able to continue.

Lighter activities

Try to build them into your normal day's activities. Try to fit a 30-minute walk in before and/or after work by getting off the bus/tube a stop earlier. Take the stairs at work instead of the lift or escalator. Leave your desk for a 5-minute walk once a day – even this little bit of exercise is estimated to reduce your body fat by two pounds annually! If you can manage a longer lunchtime walk (or maybe a swim?), even better. What about an active evening class such as salsa dancing or badminton or aqua-robics at your local pool.

Drink up, it's good for you

Drinking plenty of water is not just good for preventing heat exhaustion during exercise, but is good for the complexion and the best drink for quenching thirst. Unlike sugary fizzy drinks, it will not harm your teeth and you can use water to dilute unsweetened fruit juice. You should drink about six to eight cups/mugs/glasses of liquid a day. Replacing some/all cola drinks, tea or coffee with water will also prevent you losing vitamins through the diuretic effect of these drinks. (Diuretics make you go to the loo more often with consequent loss of water-soluble vitamins.)

Week 3

Swimming

A great exercise for women because it can be continued into pregnancy. For those not used to exercise, swimming is also easier on the heart, which does not have to pump against gravity. The water also provides body support. However, for it to be effective you need to be able to swim for half an hour.

This week, aim for 15 minutes' swimming. Make up the time with 15-minute pool exercises or a brisk walk to the pool or do some exercises when you get home. At the pool, swim two 25-metre lengths, alternating with two different strokes, if possible. Rest for a minute and repeat three times. Gradually increase the number of lengths each time you visit the pool until you are able to swim for 30 minutes.

Pool exercises

3 Water-jogging – run on the spot, bringing your knees as high as you can. Start with 20 steps per leg and build it up. 2 Water-jumps – stand in the shallow end, crouch down by bending your knees, touch the bottom of the pool then jump out of the water as high as possible. Do ten times and build it up.

Week 4

Exercise

You should be well on your way to reaching your goals, with either three aerobic sessions a week or five daily sessions of lighter aerobic activities. If you feel like a change, or are unenthusiastic about the activities you have tried so far, have a go at power walking. It can be done for free and needs nothing more than a reasonable pair of aerobic/running/cross-trainer shoes.

Power Walking

1 Walk briskly for 5 minutes. 2 Jog for 1 minute, then walk for 1 minute. Repeat ten times. 3 Walk for 15 minutes (adding short jogs, if you like). 4 Do cool-down stretches.

There are many benefits to walking. It strengthens the heart, muscles and bones, improves circulation and inspires creative thinking. Successful walkers cruise comfortably at 3.5 mph (a 17-minute mile)

Recipes

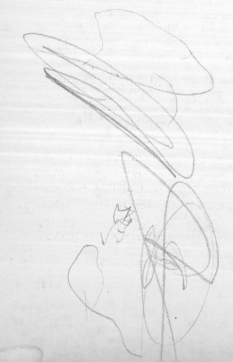

Days 1 and 15

Muesli (Hazelnut)

4 portions (store in airtight container)

4tbsp rolled oats
2tbsp chopped hazelnuts
1 ½tbsp sunflower seeds

To serve (per portion)
150ml apple juice
½ eating apple, grated

Mix the dry ingredients and place quarter in the cereal bowl. Stir in the apple juice and leave in the fridge, or a cool place, overnight. In the morning, stir in the grated apple. Add more apple juice to taste.

Short Cut Buy a sugar-free muesli equivalent to 180 calories per portion, including milk/juice to serve.

Sweetcorn polenta with spicy tomato sauce

2 portions (freeze one portion for week 3)

75g polenta (cornmeal)
180ml cold water
300ml vegetable stock
75g sweetcorn (canned with no added salt or sugar), drained or thawed if frozen
3tbsp grated Parmesan cheese
1tbsp olive oil

Blend the polenta with the water in a bowl. Bring the stock to the boil in a saucepan and add the polenta mixture in one go. Stir over a moderate heat until the mixture boils and thickens. Reduce the heat, add the sweetcorn and simmer for 10 min, until very thick, stirring to prevent sticking. Remove the pan from the heat and mix in the cheese. Spoon the mixture on to a lightly oiled baking sheet, making approx. 10cm/4in square, and smooth the top. Leave until cold, then cut into squares or wedges, lightly brush the top with oil and fry or grill for 3–4 min until golden.

Cook's Tip Choose quick-cooking polenta.

Spicy tomato sauce

4 portions (make up a quantity and freeze)

½ onion, chopped
1 clove garlic, crushed
1 red chilli, de-seeded and chopped
1tbsp fresh thyme
6 halves of sun-dried tomatoes, drained and chopped
1tbsp olive oil
400g can tomatoes

Lightly fry the onion, garlic, chilli, thyme and sun-dried tomatoes into the oil for 10 min. Add the canned tomatoes and continue to cook for 15 min until the sauce has reduced and thickened. Put the sauce in a blender or food processor and purée until smooth.

Short Cut For an extra quick, no-cook, spicy sauce, add chilli powder and crushed sun-dried tomatoes to Passata (sieved tomatoes).

Days 2 and 16

Chicken risotto

2 portions (freeze 1 for week 3)

15ml/1tbsp olive oil
1 garlic clove, crushed
½ onion, chopped
1 stick celery, chopped
225g skinless chicken, shredded
115g risotto (Italian arborio) rice
pinch saffron strands or ground turmeric, optional
300ml vegetable bouillon or chicken stock
2tbsp Parmesan, freshly grated

Heat the oil in a large, heavy-based pan and sauté the garlic, onion and celery for 10 min until softened. Add the chicken and rice and cook for 5 min, stirring to prevent sticking. Add the saffron/turmeric and stir in some of the stock. Simmer for 20 min, stirring occasionally and adding more stock until the rice has absorbed it all and is cooked. Stir in the Parmesan and serve.

Vegetable risotto

2 portions (freeze 1 portion for week 3)

15g dried mushrooms (e.g. porcini, morelles, cepes, champignon) or 50g
    fresh mushrooms
1tbsp olive oil
1 garlic clove, crushed
1 small onion, chopped
1 red pepper, diced
1 green pepper, sliced
2 sticks celery, chopped
115g risotto (Italian arborio) rice
pinch saffron strands or ground turmeric, optional
450ml vegetable bouillon or chicken stock
25g Parmesan, freshly grated

Soak the dried mushrooms (if using) in freshly boiled water, to cover
generously, for 15–20 min. Heat the oil in a large, heavy-based pan and sauté
the garlic, onion, peppers and celery for 10 min, until softened. Stir in the
rice and cook for 5 min, stirring to prevent sticking. Add the saffron/turmeric
and pour on the strained mushroom-soaking water and the stock. Simmer
for 20 min or until the rice is cooked. Stir in the Parmesan and serve.

Baked apple with date stuffing

For the stuffing, either cook 25g dried dates (about 10) in approx. 3tbsp
apple juice in a jug in a microwave for 2 min on full power, or until soft
enough to mash to a purée. Or soak the dates, then mash. Fill the apple
when cooked.

Days 3 and 17

Porridge

Make with 25g rolled oats mixed with 150ml skimmed milk and cooked
over a moderate heat, stirring all the time until thickened.

Quick porridge
Put oats and milk in a microwave dish or jug and cook on full power for 2
min, stirring once or twice. Thin with more milk, if liked. Sweeten with
1tsp honey or molasses, if liked.

Tomato soup

2 portions (freeze 1 portion for week 3)

75g split red lentils
½tsp fresh thyme
½ red pepper, roasted
225g ripe tomatoes, skinned
300ml vegetable stock
150ml semi-skimmed milk
chopped parsley to garnish, optional

Wash and pick over the lentils. Boil in twice their volume of water with the thyme for 20 min. Drain. Add the pepper and the chopped tomatoes and the stock, cover tightly and simmer until the pepper is soft, then add the milk and let the soup heat through without boiling for another minute. Garnish with the parsley.

Cook's Tip To roast a pepper, halve and deseed and place cut side down under a hot grill until the skin blisters and blackens. When cool enough to handle, peel off skin.

Avocado and pasta salad

1 portion

150g fresh pasta or 50g dry pasta
2tsp pesto
½ avocado, sliced
1 courgette, steamed and sliced
1 tomato, sliced
6 olives
60g (half a pack) mozzarella cheese, sliced

Boil the pasta until al dente (cooked but offering some resistance when bitten). Drain and toss in the pesto. Place pasta in serving dish and arrange the other salad ingredients on top.

Raisin pancake

Makes 6

50g white flour
50g wholemeal flour
1tsp bicarbonate of soda
½tsp baking powder

½tsp ground cinnamon
1 egg, lightly beaten
210ml skimmed milk soured with a few drops of lemon juice
1tbsp honey
75g raisins

Mix the flours, bicarbonate of soda, baking powder and cinnamon in a bowl. Make a well in the flour and add the egg. Gradually work in the flour from the sides of the well, adding the milk as you do so. Transfer to a food processor and whisk in the honey. Leave to stand for 30 min. Brush a non-stick pan with oil and add a ladleful of batter. Sprinkle on some raisins. Cook over a moderate heat for 2–3 min on one side, flip over and cook for 1 min on the other side.

Days 4 and 18

Tuna jacket potato

200g baked potato filled with 75g tuna in water, drained, mixed with 75g low-fat soft cheese.

Cheese jacket potato

200g baked potato filled with 25g grated cheddar mixed with ½ grated carrot and 1tbsp raisins.

Anchovy pasta

2 portions (freeze 1 portion for week 3)

1tbsp vegetable oil
½ onion, chopped
1 carrot, diced
½ red pepper, deseeded and chopped
1 courgette, sliced
400g can tomatoes, chopped
50g can anchovy fillets, drained
115g wholewheat penne (pasta)

Heat the oil in a pan and add the onion, carrot, pepper and courgettes. Cover and cook over a low heat for 15 min. Add the tomatoes and cook, uncovered, for 15 min. Meanwhile boil the pasta in plenty of water for 12–15 min. Stir the anchovies into the tomato sauce and heat through. Drain the pasta and toss in the sauce. Garnish with chopped parsley.

Spinach Gnocchi with tomato sauce

2 portions (freeze 1 portion for week 3)

175g potatoes, boiled and mashed while warm with 60ml skimmed milk
25g unbleached flour
1 free-range egg
2tbsp Parmesan, grated
115g spinach, fresh and cooked or defrosted if frozen

Beat together the potatoes, flour, egg, cheese and spinach. Form into 8 balls.
Take one portion of the tomato sauce, put in an ovenproof dish and add the
gnocchi. Bake in a preheated oven for 25 min at 190°C/375°F/Gas mark 5,
or cook in an open pan for 15 min and finish under a hot grill.

Tomato sauce

2 portions

½ onion, chopped
200g can tomatoes, chopped
1tsp tomato purée
1tbsp chopped fresh parsley
150ml vegetable stock

Sweat the onion without added fat, in a covered non-stick, or heavy-based,
pan, for about 10 min until softened. Add the tomato, tomato purée and
stock and cook for 10 min. Cool, separate into portions and use or store.

Short-cut tomato sauce
Instead of making the above tomato sauce, stir the parsley into 250ml Passata
(sieved tomatoes) available in cans and jars.

Batch cooking
You will also need tomato sauce for Meatballs/Nutballs in Tomato Sauce,
days 6/20, so why not make enough today?

Instant fruit fool

1 portion

50g no-need-to-soak dried fruit (e.g. apricots, prunes, pears)
50g Greek yogurt
50g natural yogurt

Put all the ingredients in a food processor, or press through a sieve, to produce a purée.

Days 5 and 18

Haddock and prawn fishcake

Makes 2 (freeze 1 for week 3)

175g white fish (e.g. haddock, cod, coley)
1 bay leaf
3 peppercorns
parsley stalks
50g peeled cooked prawns, chopped
115g boiled potatoes, mashed
15g dry wholemeal flour/breadcrumbs for coating
½tbsp vegetable oil for frying

Poach the fish in enough water to cover with the bay leaf, peppercorns and parsley stalks. Remove from cooking liquid and flake fish from bones. Mix the fish with the prawns and potato. Form into 2 fishcakes, using floured hands, and coat with seasoned flour. Lightly fry the fishcakes in the oil for 4–5 min each side, then drain on absorbent kitchen paper. Grill them if you do not want to use any oil.

Cook's Tip If you find it difficult forming the fishcakes while the mixture is soft and warm, allow to cool, then refrigerate and handle when cold. Cooking time will take longer from cold.

Vegetable burger

Makes 2 (freeze 1 for week 3)

175g potato, boiled
25g cheese, grated
30ml skimmed milk
50g broccoli, chopped and steamed
50g sweetcorn, drained
½ carrot, grated
1tbsp wholemeal breadcrumbs

Mash the drained potatoes with the cheese and milk. Stir in the prepared broccoli, carrot and sweetcorn. Season to taste. Divide into four and form into burgers. Roll in the breadcrumbs and grill for 12–14 min, turning once.

Cook's Tip If you find it difficult forming the burgers while the mixture is soft and warm, allow to cool, then refrigerate and handle when cold. Cooking time will take longer from cold.

Blackberry and apple summer pudding

2 portions (freeze 1 for week 3)

4 slices wholemeal bread from medium sandwich loaf, crusts removed
115g eating apples, peeled, cored and cut into chunks
115g blackberries
2tbsp water

Line the base and sides of two individual ramekins with 3 slices of bread cut to fit. Put the apples, blackberries and water in a pan, cover and cook gently for 10 min until just cooked, but not mushy. Remove from heat. Drain the fruit and transfer to the lined basin. Place the remaining slices of bread on top as a lid. Cover with greaseproof paper, then place a saucer on top and weight it so the fruit juice soaks into the bread. When cold, transfer to the fridge and chill for 2 hours, preferably overnight. To serve, invert on to a serving plate.

Days 6 and 20

Carrot and raisin muffin

Makes 10. Either make and freeze those not required for the diet, or buy equivalent wholemeal muffins, approx. 180 calories each

200g white flour
3tsp baking powder
1tsp cinnamon
50g muscovado sugar
115g raisins
1 carrot, grated
2 eggs
45ml/3tbsp sunflower oil
120ml skimmed milk

Sift the flour, baking powder and cinnamon into a bowl and stir in the sugar, raisins and carrot, making sure the raisins and carrot are coated with dry ingredients to stop them sticking together. Lightly beat the eggs, oil and milk and stir into the dry ingredients. Line a muffin pan with 10 paper muffin cases and spoon in the batter. Bake in a preheated oven at 190°C/375°/Gas mark 5 for 20–25 minutes or until well risen and an inserted skewer comes out clean.

Meatballs in tomato sauce

2 portions (freeze 1 for week 3)

225g lean meat (e.g. chicken, rabbit, venison, pigeon)
40g pine kernels
1 onion, quartered
1 carrot, chopped
2tsp chopped fresh herbs (e.g. tarragon or thyme with rabbit, sage with
    venison, rosemary)
1tsp mild ready-made mustard

Put the meat in a food processor. Lightly toast the pine kernels, turning once or twice for 10 min in a moderate oven or under a grill. Add the pine kernels and the rest of the ingredients to the processor and blend to desired consistency. Form into meatballs, dusting with a little seasoned flour and cook in Tomato sauce (see Gnocchi recipe, day 4) either in a pan on the hob for 20 min, or in a medium oven 190°C/375°/Gas mark 5 for 20–25 min.

Nutballs in tomato sauce

2 portions (freeze one for week 3)

40g hazelnuts, ground
40g walnuts, finely chopped
40g wholemeal flour
40g pine kernels
1 onion, grated
1 carrot, grated
1 egg
1tsp garam masala

Substitute the nuts for the meat in the meatballs recipe and follow the instructions.

Days 7 and 21

Mediterranean vegetable pie

Makes 2 (freeze 1 for week 3)

1 aubergine
75g green beans
½ red pepper
½ × 115g pack filo pastry
25g unsalted butter, melted
125g pack half-fat mozzarella cheese, sliced
115g can pinto beans

Dice the vegetables and steam until slightly softened. Line two individual pie tins with the filo pastry, brushing with butter between layers. Leave excess hanging over the edges. Mix the vegetables, beans and cheese and fill the pastry cases. Seal the tops by twisting the pastry ends together, brush with butter, and bake for 25 min at 190°C/375°F/Gas mark 5.

Apple tart

If you do not want to cook the tart, have a baked apple filled with raisins and 1tsp organic maize malt syrup or clear honey

2 portions (freeze 1 for week 3)

1 large eating apple (225g)
2tsp organic maize malt syrup or clear honey
4 sheets filo pastry (about ⅛ pack)
15g unsalted butter, melted

Peel and slice the apples and 'fry' in the syrup in a pan for 10 min. Line a small tin, or flan ring on a baking sheet, with the pastry, buttering between sheets and leaving a small amount hanging over the edges. Fill the pastry case with the drained apples. Scrunch the overlapping pastry into a 'frill' around the edge of the tin, brush the edge with butter and bake for 15 min at 190°C/375°F/Gas mark 5. Serve immediately.

Days 8 and 22

Seafood lasagne

2 portions (freeze 1 for week 4)

175g smoked or natural haddock
300ml skimmed milk
2tsp cornflour
pinch ground nutmeg
½ onion, chopped
2tsp vegetable oil
150ml Passata
Tabasco, optional
115g large peeled prawns
75g ready-to-use lasagne

Poach the haddock in enough water to cover, drain and flake the fish into chunks from the skin and remove bones. Heat most of the milk, reserving a little to mix with the cornflour. When the milk nears boiling, stir in the cornflour and thicken. Season and add nutmeg and the haddock.

While the haddock is poaching, sauté the onion in the oil for 10 min until soft. Stir in the Pasatta and season (add a dash of Tabasco, if liked). Stir in the prawns and heat through. Put a little tomato sauce in the base of an ovenproof dish and cover with a layer of lasagne. Top with half the tomato and prawn sauce. Add a layer of lasagne and then half the fish sauce. Repeat. Cover the dish with foil and bake in a preheated oven at 190°C/375°F/Gas 5 for 25–30 min, removing the foil for the last 5–10 min to lightly brown the top layer.

Cook's Note The sauces may seem sloppy but ready-to-use, or no-pre-cook lasagne, absorbs more liquid than the pre-cooked variety.

Pepper and spinach lasagne

2 portions (freeze 1 for week 4)

1 red pepper, deseeded and halved
1 yellow pepper, deseeded and halved
4 plum tomatoes, skinned and sliced
300ml Passata
Tabasco, optional
450g fresh spinach cooked, or 225g frozen, defrosted
225g medium fat soft white cheese or fromage frais
½tsp ground nutmeg
75g ready-to-use lasagne

Flatten the pepper halves and put under a hot grill until they are charred and blistered. When cool enough to handle, remove the skin and slice into strips. Mix in a bowl with the tomatoes and Pasatta and season (adding a dash of Tabasco, if liked). Mix the spinach, fromage frais and nutmeg and season well. Layer and cook the dish as described for Seafood lasagne.

Days 9 and 23

Chicken stir-fry

2 portions (freeze 1 for week 4)

2tsp vegetable oil
1 garlic clove, crushed
1cm root ginger, peeled and grated
225g skinless chicken, shredded
1 carrot, cut into matchsticks
50g broccoli florets
1 red pepper, de-seeded and cut into strips
1 onion, sliced
115g mangetout, trimmed

Heat the oil in a wok or large, heavy-based frying pan. Add the garlic, ginger and chicken and stir-fry until garlic is almost softened, but not browned (this will make the garlic bitter). Add the vegetables and stir-fry over a high heat for 4 min, or until the vegetables are cooked to your taste. Add some Sweet and sour sauce for extra flavour.

Quorn stir-fry

Omit the chicken and use instead 325g unflavoured chunks of Quorn, which is added along with the vegetables. Pour on Sweet and sour sauce after the first 2 min of cooking and allow the dish to finish cooking in it.

Freezing Tip Freeze the stir-fries in Sweet and sour sauce.

Sweet and sour sauce

2 portions (freeze 1 for week 4)

1 ½tbsp shoyu or soy sauce
juice of ½ orange
1tsp tomato purée
2tsp white wine vinegar

2tsp demerara sugar
1tsp cornflour mixed with 2tbsp cold water

Heat the sauce ingredients, except cornflour, in a pan over a moderate heat, stirring constantly until the sugar has dissolved. Stir in the cornflour mixture and cook until the sauce has slightly thickened.

Fruit crunch

½ Jordans Crunchy bar, or similar, crushed
115g apple purée (or babyfood fruit purée)
115g low-fat fromage frais or yogurt

Swirl all the ingredients together in an individual serving dish.

Days 10 and 24

Waldorf salad

½ eating apple, peeled and chopped
1 celery stick, chopped
25g walnut pieces

Yogurt dressing
2 tbsp natural yogurt
squeeze of lemon juice
freshly ground black pepper

Toss the apple, celery and walnut in the dressing.

Mackerel kebabs

1 medium mackerel fillet, skinned
110g coley fillet, skinned
½tsp ground cumin
½tsp ground coriander
pinch of ground turmeric
1tsp tomato purée

Put the fish in a food processor with the spices and tomato purée and blend to a smooth purée. Divide the mixture in half; with floured hands, carefully form around 2 skewers. Preheat the grill and put the kebabs on an oiled sheet of cooking foil and cook for 5 minutes each side, turning carefully.

Nut shish kebabs

Blend as for Nutballs, then shape in same way as Mackerel kebabs (days 10 and 24).

Days 11 and 25

Salsa (Mexican hot sauce)

2 portions (1 portion for vegetarians, day 11)

1 red chilli, halved and de-seeded
½ red pepper, halved and de-seeded
1 garlic clove
2 plum tomatoes, skinned
squeeze of lime juice
15g pack coriander, finely chopped

Flatten the chilli and pepper halves with the heel of your hand and put under a hot grill, skin side uppermost, until charred and black. When cool enough to handle, remove the skin and put in a food processor with the garlic, tomatoes and lime juice. Blend to a purée and stir in the coriander. Store in the fridge until ready to use.

WARNING Wear rubber gloves when handling chillies to avoid chilli 'burns' when touching eyes and other sensitive areas.

Short Cut If buying salsa, choose approx. 30 cals/serving.

Calzone (pizza turnover)

Makes 2 (freeze 1 for week 4)

50g wholemeal flour
115g unbleached white flour
½ sachet Easybake yeast
75ml water at 43°C/110°F
60g half-fat mozzarella
50g mushrooms
2 plum tomatoes, sliced
1tsp tomato purée
1tsp chopped fresh herbs

Mix the flours and yeast in a bowl. Stir in the water and knead the dough for 10 min. Cover and leave in a draught-free place to double in size.

Alternatively, speed proving by putting dough in an oiled bowl and micro-waving on full power for 10 sec., rest for 10 min. Repeat twice. Knead again and roll into a 12cm/5in square. Cut into half. Spread the dough with tomato purée, leaving 2.5cm/1in around the edges. Sprinkle on herbs and place the filling (mushrooms, tomatoes, cheese) in a triangle shape. Moisten the edges with water or egg wash and fold over, pinching to seal. Brush the top with egg wash and sprinkle over flour in a lattice pattern. Bake for 15 min at 425°C/220°F/Gas mark 7.

Coeur à la crème

1 portion

40g reduced-fat Greek yogurt
75g low fat soft white cheese
1 egg white
115g berries (e.g. blackberries, raspberries, strawberries)

Beat together the yogurt and cheese. Whisk the egg white until it forms a stiff peak and fold 2tbsp into the cheese mixture. Carefully fold in the rest and spoon into two heart-shaped Coeur à la crème ceramic moulds, lined with butter muslin. Stand in the fridge on a tray or plate to catch the drips for at least two hours. Purée the fruit and press through a sieve to make a sauce.

Cook's Tip If you have no Coeur à la crème moulds, use yogurt pots punctured with a skewer.

Days 12 and 26

Black bean and corn soup

Serves 2 (freeze 1 for week 4)

75g black beans
1 small onion, chopped
1 red pepper, de-seeded and chopped
1 chilli, de-seeded and chopped
1 garlic clove, crushed
½tsp fresh thyme leaves
1tbsp olive oil
450ml vegetable stock
200g can tomatoes
115g sweetcorn kernels canned without added water or sugar

Soak the beans in boiling water for 2 hours. Drain and boil in a saucepan with plenty of water for 10 min. Reduce heat and cook for 1 hour, topping up the water as necessary. Sauté the onion, pepper, chilli, garlic and thyme in the oil for 5 min. Add half the stock and cook until the onions and peppers are soft. Put the tomatoes and their juice, the remaining stock, the beans and onion mixture in a food processor and purée. For a smoother soup, press all or most of it through a sieve or mouli. Return to a clean pan and cook for 15 min. Add the corn kernels and heat through.

Rösti

1 portion

1 medium potato, grated
½ leek, chopped
115g canned or cooked pinto beans, drained
1tsp vegetable oil

Mix the potato, leek and beans. Heat half the oil in a pan and add the vegetable mixture, forming into a cake. Fry on one side for 7–8 min, carefully turn and cook the other side for 2–3 min. Serve with a mixed green salad (no dressing).

Trifle

150ml low fat custard (ready-made or home-made with skimmed milk)
¼ jelly
2 boudoir biscuits (sponge fingers) or 4 ratafias
115g chopped fruit of choice (if canned, in juice, not syrup)

Make the jelly and pour over the fruit and broken biscuits, or ratafia, in the bottom of an individual serving dish. Leave to set and pour over the custard.

Days 13 and 27

Savoury breakfast croissant

Makes 8 (freeze 6, 1 needed for day 14)

225g unbleached flour
50g each wholemeal flour and polenta (maize flour)
1 sachet EasyBake yeast
150ml buttermilk (or milk soured with a few drops of lemon juice)
1tbsp sunflower oil

25g matured cheddar, grated
40ml water, optional
40g pine kernels or sunflower seeds, lightly toasted

Mix the flours in a bowl and stir in the yeast. Warm the buttermilk to 43°C/110°F and stir into the flour with the oil and cheddar. Knead on a floured surface for 10 min. If the dough seems dry, add the water, warmed to the same temperature as the milk. Place in a bowl and cover. Leave in a draught-free warm place for 40 min to double in size. Knead again for 2 min, working in the pine kernels/sunflower seeds. Shape by rolling the dough into a circle and cutting into eight triangles. Roll each triangle into a croissant shape, starting from the outer edge of the circle and rolling towards the point. Put on a greased baking tray. Cover and leave as before for 30 min until double in size. Brush with milk and bake for 15 min at 200°C/400°F/Gas mark 6.

Bruschetta

2 slices ciabatta
1tsp tomato purée
1tsp chopped fresh basil
½ pepper, de-seeded and chopped
¼ onion, chopped
4 cherry tomatoes, halved
50g firm goat's cheese

Toast the bread on one side, turn over and top with the tomato purée mixed with the basil. Spread over the vegetables and sliced cheese and return to the grill until the cheese is melted to desired consistency. Serve with mixed green salad (no dressing).

NB If preferred, lightly cook the onion, pepper and tomatoes before topping the toast.

Scotch egg

1 portion

½ onion, grated
25g medium oatmeal
25g ground hazelnuts
1tbsp tomato purée
3tbsp boiling water
1 egg, hard-boiled and shelled
egg wash or milk
1tbsp dry wholemeal breadcrumbs

Put the onion, oatmeal, hazelnuts, tomato purée and water in a bowl/food processor and blend to a thick paste. With floured hands mould the paste around the egg. Dip in egg wash and roll in breadcrumbs. Bake on a lightly oiled baking sheet for 20 min, turning once during cooking, at 190°C/ 375°F/Gas mark 5. Cool and refrigerate until ready for use.

Warm fruit brûlée

1 portion

115g blackberries
4 ready-to-eat prunes, chopped
100ml half-fat crème fraîche
12g fructose (fruit sugar) or demerara sugar

Warm the berries in a pan with a couple of tablespoonsful of water until the juices begin to run. Add the prunes and then transfer to an individual ramekin or similar ovenproof dish. Top with the crème fraîche and sprinkle over the sugar. Put under a hot grill until the sugar bubbles and caramelizes.

Days 14 and 28

Rabbit/chicken casserole

2 portions (freeze 1 for week 4)

300g boned and cubed rabbit/chicken
1tbsp flour, seasoned
1tbsp vegetable oil
1 large eating apple, peeled and sliced
2 sticks celery, chopped
75g mushrooms, sliced

Toss the meat in seasoned flour and lightly brown in half the oil. Remove the meat from the pan and put on one side. Add the rest of the ingredients and mix well. Cover the pan and cook over a low heat for 15 min to soften the vegetables.

Return the meat to the pan with just enough water to cover and any flour. Cover and cook over a medium heat, stirring occasionally, for 15 min.

Minestrone casserole

2 portions (freeze 1 for week 4)

75g green beans, sliced
2 courgettes, sliced
2 carrots, sliced
4 baby new potatoes
vegetable stock or water
115g macaroni
400g can cannellini beans

*Pesto Sauce**
15g fresh basil, chopped
2 tomatoes, skinned
1 garlic clove
1tbsp olive oil
seasoning

Put the beans, courgettes, carrots and potatoes in a pan and cover with stock or water. Simmer for 15 min. Add the macaroni and top up with water or stock and simmer for 20 min. Stir in the beans and heat through for 10 min. To make the sauce, put the ingredients in a food processor and blend to a purée. Stir the sauce into the casserole at the end of cooking and heat through.
* Use 1tbsp bought pesto, if preferred.

Selected Bibliography

Reports, papers and miscellaneous

1 The National Food Guide, The Balance of Good Health (1994), Health Education Authority in partnership with the Department of Health and the Ministry of Agriculture, Fisheries and Food

2 Diet, nutrition and the prevention of chronic diseases (1990), report of a World Health Organization Study Group

3 Nutritional Aspects of Coronary Heart Disease (1994), report of Committee on Medical Aspects of Food Policy

4 Dietary Reference Values for Food Energy and Nutrients for the UK (1991), report of the panel on Dietary Reference Values of the Committee on Medical Aspects of Food Policy

5 Physical Activity Strategy Statement (1996), Physical Activity Task Force, Department of Health

6 Medical Aspects of Exercise, Benefits and Risks (1991), report of the Royal College of Physicians

7 Allied Dunbar National Fitness Survey (1993), in conjunction with the Health Education Authority, Sports Council and Look After Your Heart

8 The Use of Very Low Calorie Diets in Obesity (1987), report of the Working Group on Very Low Calorie Diets, Committee on Medical Aspects of Food Policy, Department of Health and Social Security

9 Obesity (1983), a report of the Royal College of Physicians

10 Obesity, Reversing the Increasing Problem of Obesity in England (1995), a report from The Nutrition and Physical Activity Task Forces, The Health of the Nation

11 Exploding the Myths of Obesity (1995) symposium organized by the Association for the Study of Obesity, St Bartholomew's Hospital, London

12 The Health of the Nation (1992) a strategy for health in England

13 Why we eat what we eat (1990), The British Nutrition Foundation *Nutrition Bulletin* 15, supplement 1

14 A role for glucagon-like peptide-1 in the central regulation of feeding, *Nature*, Vol. 379, 69–72

15 Don't blame the metabolism (1995), Andrew Prentice, *Medical Research Council News*, Autumn, 27–33

16 Food Choice (1994), Institute of Food Research annual report

17 Cognitive Effects of Diet, presented by Dr Michael Green and Dr Peter Rogers of the Institute of Food Research at a London meeting of the British Psychological Society, 15 December 1992
18 Measuring Sensory Quality, Dr David Kilcast, Leatherhead Research Association
19 *The Natural History Programme*, BBC Radio 4, 19 September 1995

Books

20 *The Complete Guide to Homeopathy* (1995), Dr Andrew Lockie and Dr Nicola Geddes (Dorling Kindersley)
21 *The Driving Force, Food, Evolution and the Future* (1989), Michael Crawford and David Marsh (Heinemann)
22 *Eat for Life Diet* (1992), Janette Marshall and Anne Heughan (Vermilion)
23 *Eating Disorders and Obesity* (1995), editors K.D. Brownell and C.G. Fairburn (Guildford Press, London)
24 *Evolution and Healing, the New Science of Darwinian Medicine* (1995), Randolph M. Nesse and George C. Williams (Weidenfeld & Nicolson)
25 *The Family Guide to Homeopathy* (1989), Dr Andrew Lockie (Hamish Hamilton)
26 *Healthy Eating on a Plate* (1995), Janette Marshall (Vermilion)
27 *Obesity and Related Disorders* (1988), J.S. Garrow (Churchill Livingstone)
28 *The Ultimate Ace Diet* (1994), Janette Marshall (Vermilion)
29 *The Women's Guide to Homeopathy* (1992), Dr Andrew Lockie and Dr Nicola Geddes (Hamish Hamilton)

Useful Addresses

Societies and Organizations

Faculty of Homeopathy
The Royal London Homeopathic Hospital
Great Ormond Street
London WC1N 3HR
(provides a list of medically qualified homeopaths).

The British Homeopathic Association
27a Devonshire Street
London W1N 1RJ
(provides a list of medically qualified homeopaths).

The Homeopathic Society
2 Powis Place
Great Ormond Street
London WC1N 3HT
(provides a list of medically qualified homeopaths).

The Society of Homeopaths
2 Artizan Road
Northampton NN1 4HU
(provides a register of non-medically qualified homeopaths).

NHS Homeopathic Hospitals

Homeopathic doctors working within the National Health Service can refer patients to:

Bristol Homeopathic Hospital
Cotham Hill
Cotham
Bristol BS6 6JU

Department of Homeopathic Medicine
Mossley Hill Hospital
Park Avenue
Liverpool L I 8 8BU

Glasgow Homeopathic Hospital
1000 Great Western Road
Glasgow G I 2 0ET

Royal London Homeopathic Hospital
Great Ormond Street
London WC I N 3HR

Tunbridge Wells Homeopathic Hospital
Church Road
Tunbridge Wells
Kent TN I I JU

Suppliers of Homeopathic Remedies

Most chemists and health food stores stock a limited range of homeopathic
remedies. The following specialist pharmacies or manufacturers stock a full
range of remedies. All will supply products by post.

Ainsworths Pharmacy
36 New Cavendish Street
London W I M 7LH

Buxton and Grant
176 Whiteladies Road
Bristol BS8 2XU

Freeman's Pharmacy
7 Eaglesham Road
Clarkston
Glasgow G76 7BU

Galen Homeopathics
Lewell Mill
W. Stafford
Dorchester
Dorset DT2 8AN

Goulds the Chemist
14 Crowndale Road
London NW1 1TT

Helios Pharmacy
97 Camden Road
Tunbridge Wells
Kent TN1 2QR

A. Nelson & Co. Ltd
73 Duke Street
London W1M 6BY

Weleda (UK) Ltd (licensed manufacturer)
Heanor Road
Ilkeston
Derbyshire DE7 8DR

Biochemic Tissue Salts and Combination Remedies

New Era Laboratories Ltd,
Marfleet
Hedon Road
Kingston-upon-Hull HU9 5NJ

Bach Flower Remedies

Dr Edward Bach Centre
Mount Vernon
Sotwell
Wallingford
Oxon OX10 0PZ

Homeopathic Equipment

Phials, storage bottles, unmedicated tablets and other homeopathic supplies can be obtained by post from:

Trevor Cook, (Homeopathy) Ltd
Victor House
Norris Road
Staines
Middlesex TW18 4DS

The Homeopathic Supply Co.
4 Nelson Road
Sheringham
Norfolk NR26 8BU

General Index

active lifestyle, 39–42
advertising foodstuffs, 6
aerobics, *see* exercise
alcohol,
    calorie content, 100
    low-risk levels, 49
    moderate drinking, 48–9
    see also drink
alpha-linolenic fatty acid, 46
anaemia, 51
anchovy pasta, 153
anorexia, 118
antioxidant minerals, 51
appearance of food, 15
appetite,
    appetite-suppressant pills, 12, 111
    how it works, 11
    natural, *see* natural appetite
    restraining, 5
    stimulating, 13–14
    Stone Age, 3–4
    see also natural appetite
apple tart, 158
arrhythmia, 10
Arsenicum album (Ars.), 134
avocado and pasta salad, 152

baked apple with date stuffing, 151
BMI units, 7
beans, 51–2
black bean and corn soup, 163
blackberry and apple summer
    pudding, 156
beauty therapists, 113
blood-sugar levels, 12, 13, 16
Body Mass Index (BMI),

calculation, 43–4
gene responsible for, 7, 107
male reluctance to acknowledge
    problem, 110–11
body shapes, 4–5, 8
brain,
    and appetite, 12
    chemicals, 14
    dieting's effect on, 10–11
bread, 33–4, 36
    in Natural Diet, 56
    sandwiches, 56
breakfast, 32–3, 57
bruschetta, 165
bulimia, 118
butter or margarine?, 46–7

Calcarea (Calc.), 130
calcium, 37
calories,
    burning off, 7, 32
    content of drinks, 100
    daily intake, 9
    eating more than expending, 8
    experience regulating intake,
        16–17
    in fats, 45–6
    high-calorie foods, 3
    positive/negative energy balance,
        4
    shopping lists for 1,200 calorie
        diet, 62–74
calzone (pizza turnover), 162
cancer, 51
carbohydrates
    energy from, 5

suppressant for sweet food, 35
    see also bread; cereals; potatoes
carrot and raisin muffin, 156
Causticum (Caust.), 135
cellulite-reducing creams, 113
cereals, 33–4, 36, 51–2
cheese jacket potato, 153
chewing, 14
chicken,
    risotto, 150
    stir-fry, 160
child-bearing, effect of, 107–8
chocolate addiction, 14, 109
cholesterol, 45
coeur à la crème, 163
comfort food, 13
composite foods, 38–9
cravings, 14, 141
Cushing's Syndrome, 117

dental problems, 47–8
depression, 14
diet,
    balanced, 33–6
    eating between meals, 33–4
    hunter-gatherers' variety, 31
    maintenance, 142–3
    today's limited diet, 32
    see also natural appetite; natural
        diet; slimming diet
Doctrine of Signatures, 22
dowsing, 26
drinks,
    calorie content, 100
    and exercise, 147
    fruit juice, 57
    in Natural Diet, 56
    see also alcohol
drugs controlling appetite, 12

eggs, 51, 57
emotions, 129
energy,
    from carbohydrates, 36
    from foods of different human
        groups, 5
    loss of, 115
    positive/negative energy balance,
        4, 45
evening meals, 33
exercise,
    activity level scale, 42
    adverse effects of, 9
    aerobics, 39–42, 113, 145, 146
    combined with diet, 8
    and drinking, 147
    four-week maintenance activity
        plan, 145–9
    lighter activities, 43, 147
    moderate activity, 42
    overdoing, 146
    power walking, 149
    and smoking, 149
    sustaining weight loss, 144
    swimming and pool exercises,
        148
    target levels, 42
    vigorous activity, 43
    warming up and cooling down,
        146

Faculty of Homeopathy, 137
fatty foods,
    butter or margarine?, 46–7
    calories in, 45–6
    energy from, 5
    essential fatty acids, 31, 46, 51
    natural appetite for, 3–4
    over-eating, 16
    portions, 38
    satiety and, 16
    saturated, polyunsaturates and
        monounsaturates, 45–6, 50
    underestimating intake, 114
fibre,
    energy from, 5

giving full feeling, 48
high-fibre foods, 35, 51
fish,
 oily, 46
 portions, 37
 white fish, 51
Food Diary, 55
food types,
 strong likes, 124–5
 strong dislikes, 126
 aggravations, 127–8
 charts, 122–3
 food information, 122–3
fruit, 33–4, 36–7
fruit crunch, 161

GLP-1 (glucagon-like peptide 1),
 12
genetic make-up,
 environmental influences, 8
 failure to pass on healthy genes,
  32
 inherited proneness to put on
  weight, 6–7
 misconceptions about, 107
 obesity gene, 7, 107

Hahnemann, Samuel Christopher,
 22–5
haddock and prawn fishcake, 155
heart disease, 8, 10, 51
herbal supplements, 113
Hippocrates, 22
homeopathy,
 Cartesian split in medicine, 21–2
 Doctrine of Signatures, 22
 history of, 22
 laws of, 27–8
 low- and high-potency
  prescribers, 25–6
 and natural appetite, 26–8
 paying for treatment, 138
 potentized medicines, 24, 25

practitioners, 137–8
principles of, 22
to regain natural appetite, 136
remedies
 availability of, 136
 finding right remedies, see
  food types
 further help, 137
 reactions to, 137
 storage, 136
remedy pictures, 129–35
 Arsenicum album, 134
 Calcarea, 130
 Causticum, 135
 Kali carbonicum, 134
 Lachesis, 133
 Lycopodium, 130–31
 Mercurius, 135
 Natrum muriaticum, 133–4
 Phosphorus, 132–3
 Pulsatilla, 132
 Sepia, 131
 Sulphur, 131–2
 similars, 23–4
hunger,
 cravings, 14, 141
 mouth hunger, 13–14
 physiological triggers, 11
hypnotherapy, 113
hypothyroidism, 116

influences affecting food intake, 6
instant fruit fool, 154
iron, 52

junk food, 5

Kali carbonicum (Kali, c.), 134

Lachesis (Lach.), 133
laxatives, 117
legumes, 51–2
lifestyle, 14, 23–4, 39–42, 45

liquid-meal replacements, 113
low-fat spreads, 47, 57
Lycopodium (Lyc.), 130–31

mackerel kebabs, 161
maintenance diet, 142
margarine, 57
meat,
    alternatives, 37, 50
    farmed cattle, 50
    portions, 37
    poultry, 50–51
    protein provider, 50
    saturated fats in, 50
    wild animals, 50
meatballs in tomato sauce, 157
Mediterranean vegetable pie, 158
Mercurius (Merc.), 135
metabolism,
    adjusting to Natural Diet, 115
    damaging by dieting, 9
    misconceptions about, 106
    peak metabolic rate, 33
    rate slowing during dieting, 9
milk and dairy foods, 33–4, 37, 47,
    57
minestrone casserole, 167
monounsaturates, 45
monosodium glutamate (MSG), 15
mouth hunger, 13–14
muesli (hazelnut), 149
muscle tissue, 9

Natrum muriaticum (Nat. m.), 133
natural appetite,
    adjusting, 9–10, 11–12
    in balance, 11
    controlled by brain, 12
    desynchronized by dieting, 11
    for fat, 45–6
    food groups, 34–6
    harmonizing, 14–17
    and homeopathy, 26–8, 136

inappropriateness of, 3
meaning of, 12–14
for non-slimmers, 55–6
out of balance, 15
reverting to, 32–6
for slimmers, 55
stress and, 21
see also appetite; diet; Natural
    Diet
Natural Diet,
    additional food allowance, 74
    general instructions, 56–7
    individual requirements, 35
    maintenance plan, 141–7
        cravings returning, 141
        maintenance activity plan,
            144–7
        motivation, 141–2
    menus
        basic, 58–9
        daily, 75–88
    for non-slimmers, 55–6
    portions, 36–9
    problems
        anorexia, 118
        bulimia, 118
        indigestion and bowel
            problems, 116–17
        physical, emotional and
            general changes, 129
    problems with
        energy loss, 116
        headaches, 115
        medical problems, 116–17
        unwell feeling, 115–16
    restaurant meals
        menus, 90–99
        aperitifs, 90
        starters, 90
        main course, 91
        cheese, 91
        pudding/dessert, 91
        coffee, 91

petits fours, 91
    liqueurs, 91
shopping lists for 1,200 calorie
    diet, 62–73
for slimmers, 55
store cupboard items, 60–61
negative energy balance, 4, 45
neuropeptide-Y, 12
neurotransmitters, 11
nut shish kebabs
nutballs in tomato sauce, 157
nuts and seeds, 51

obesity,
    fat distribution, 7–8
    and feminist myth, 110
    gene, 107
    health risks, 105, 110, 112
    increasing incidence of, 4
    laying down body fat, 7
    male reluctance to acknowledge
        problem, 110–11
    measuring, see Body Mass Index
    medical conditions causing, 116
    and metabolism, 106
    under-recording food intake, 106
    see also weight
Omega-3 and Omega-6, 46
oral contraceptive, 116
organic foods, 56

Paraceslus, 25
pepper and spinach lasagne, 159
Phosphorus (Phos.), 132–3
polenta, sweetcorn, 149
polyunsaturates, 45
porridge, 151
portions, 36–41
    for those not slimming, 39
potatoes, 33–4, 36
pregnant women, 46, 49, 51, 56
preserves, 57
proteins,

energy from, 5
    food providing, 35
    hormone-based drugs, 12
psionic medicine, 26
psychological feedback, 11
Pulsatilla (Puls.), 132
pulses, 51–2

quorn stir-fry, 160

rabbit/chicken casserole, 166
raisin pancake, 152
remedy pictures, see homeopathy
restaurant meals, see Natural Diet
rösti, 164

salsa (Mexican hot sauce), 162
salt, 5
satiety,
    mechanisms indicating, 16
    physiological triggers, 11
savoury breakfast croissant, 164
Scotch egg, 165
seafood lasagne, 159
sedentary lifestyle,
    and negative energy balance, 45
sedentary lifestyle, see lifestyle
Sepia (Sep.), 131
serotonin, 14
shopping lists, 56, 57
    basic 1,200 calorie, 62–73
Signatures, Doctrine of, 22
similars, 23
slimming clubs, 111
slimming diets,
    brain, effect on, 10–11
    calorie intake required, 9
    chronic (yo-yo), 9, 114
    crash diets: medical risks, 9–10
    desynchronizing natural appetite,
        11
    essential nutrients, 10
    and exercise combined, 8

failure of, 9
loss of muscle tissue, 9
meal replacement, 10
painless, 112−13
regaining lost weight, 4−5, 9
slow weight loss, 111−12
spot-reduction, 8
starvation response, 9
wrong types of, 113
see also Natural Diet
smoking, 8, 109−10, 149
snacks, 13, 33
Society of Homeopaths, 138
spicy tomato sauce, 150
spinach gnocchi with tomato sauce,
  154
starchy food, 16
starvation response, 9
steroids, 116
Stone Age diet, 3−4, 31
stress, 21, 108−9
sugar,
  artificial sweeteners, 35
  chocolate addiction, 14, 108
  energy from, 5
  excessive consumption of, 47−8
  natural appetite for, 3−4, 13−14
  portions of sugary foods, 38
  sweets and confectionery, 33−4,
    48
Sulphur (Sulph.), 131−2
sweet and sour sauce, 160

takeaway meals,
  safety advice, 101
  swaps, 101
taste,
  based on appearance and texture,
    15

buds, 15−16
tomato soup, 152
trifle, 164
tuna jacket potato, 153

umami, 15

variety of diet, 31−2
vegetable burgers, 155
vegetable oil, 57
vegetable risotto, 151
vegetables, 33−4, 36−7
vegetarianism, 51−2, 61
Vital Force, 28

Waist to Hip Circumference Ratio
  (WHR), 7−8
Waldorf salad, 161
walking, 149
warm fruit brûlée, 166
weight,
  calculations, 43−4
  child-bearing, effect of, 107−8
  gain
    from saturated fats, 46
  slow weight loss, 111−12
  storage fat, 46
  and stress, 108−9
  see also obesity
willpower, 27−8
women,
  body shape, 8
  child-bearing, effect of, 107−8
  fat/muscle proportion, 9
  pregnancy and dieting, 46, 49,
    51, 56
  unrealistic body images, 6

yogurt, 57